U.S. GUIDE TO

VENOMOUS
Snakes
AND THEIR
MIMICS

Scott Shupe

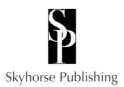

Skyhorse Publishing

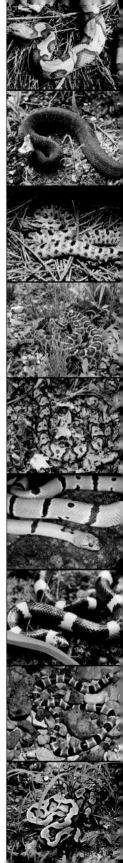

Skyhorse Publishing books may be purchased in bulk at special discounts for sales promotion, corporate gifts, fund-raising, or educational purposes. Special editions can also be created to specifications. For details, contact the Special Sales Department, Skyhorse Publishing, 307 West 36th Street, 11th Floor, New York, NY 10018 or info@skyhorsepublishing.com.

Skyhorse® and Skyhorse Publishing® are registered trademarks of Skyhorse Publishing, Inc.®, a Delaware corporation.

Visit our website at www.skyhorsepublishing.com.

10 9 8 7 6 5 4

Library of Congress Cataloging-in-Publication Data

Shupe, Scott.
US guide to venomous snakes and their mimics / by Scott Shupe.
p. cm.
Includes bibliographical references.
Hardcover ISBN 978-1-61608-182-9 (hardcover : alk. paper)
1. Poisonous snakes--United States--Identification. 2. Poisonous snakes--United States. 3. Snakes--United States--Identification. I. Title. II. Title: U.S. guide to venomous snakes and their mimics.
QL666.O6S43 2010
597.96'1650973--dc22
2010031935

Cover design by Qualcom
Cover photographs courtesy of the author

Print ISBN: 978-1-5107-4000-6
Ebook ISBN: 978-1-62873-314-3

Printed in China

CONTENTS

PREFACE

The goal of this book is to provide all those who enjoy the outdoors with a quick and reliable guide to identifying that small percentage of snakes that pose a real threat to man.

With that goal in mind, I have used color photographs in order to give a completely accurate representation of both venomous species and harmless non-venomous species that closely resemble the dangerous snake species.

While there are a number of very authoritative books available on the reptiles of the United States, most deal with animals native only to a specific area or state, or else they are so broad in scope that they are cumbersome for the average person trying to quickly and accurately identify a particular snake seen in their backyard or on a recent outdoor experience.

In writing this book, I have tried to make it as easy as possible for the average outdoors person (hunter, fisherman, backpacker, gardener, etc.) to quickly and correctly ascertain whether or not the snake in question is, in fact, a dangerous species. I have tried to achieve the goal of identification using the simple method of dividing the entire country into several regions, then providing a set of color photographs of the dangerous snakes of each region, as well as photos of similar harmless species within that region that are often confused with the dangerous species.

For the benefit of those with more than just the practical interest in identifying a particular snake, I have in the written text provided detailed information on the natural history of each species and subspecies. Much of this information is borrowed from previously published books and journals, while some of it is of a more personal, anecdotal nature. Wherever my memory served, I have included personal experiences and observations gleaned from some 40 years of hunting, studying, and observing snakes both in the wild and in captivity. In one sense, I guess, this book is for the author an attempt to justify having spent such an inordinate amount of my life in pursuit of a passion that most folks in my tiny western Kentucky hometown would politely refer to as "just a little peculiar."

In keeping with my goal of a scientifically accurate text, I have used some technical terminology in describing the physical characteristics, behavior, and natural history of each species and subspecies. For those not familiar with these terms, an alphabetically arranged glossary is provided in the back of this book.

ACKNOWLEDGEMENTS

The author wishes to express his appreciation to the following individuals and organizations who have contributed to this book. They are, in no paticular order: Jim Harrison—Kentucky Reptile Zoo, Jared Baker—Birmingham Zoo, Steve Reichling—Memphis Zoo, Dale McGinnity—Nashville Zoo, David Baum—U.S. Army Corps of Engineers at Carlyle Lake, Illinois, Carlton Burke and Bob Fay—Western North Carolina Nature Center, Joe Mairhauser, Don Middaugh, Tom Lang, and Bill Texel—Reptile Gardens, the late E. Ross Allen, the late Bill Gleason, the late Bill Phelps, and Andrew Koukoulis of the former Ross Allen Reptile Institute, David Drysdale—St. Augustine Alligator Farm, Kenny Maddox—Lake City, Florida, Tom Moxley—Memphis, Tennessee, Bob Myers—American Rattlesnake Museum, Jim Peters—Clermont, Florida, Ed Cassano-Clermont, Florida, Nancy Smith—Jones-Tucson, Arizona, John McGregor—Kentucky Department of Fish & Wildlife Resources, Dr. Ed Zimmerer—Murray State University, and Patricia and Dick Bartlett—Gainesville, Florida.

The following individuals provided the author with additional photographs for the book: Andrew Koukoulis, Dale McGinnity, Nancy Smith-Jones, Ed Cassano, and Dick Bartlett. Black and white drawings provided by Gary Lopiccolo, color drawing by James Dobson.

Thanks is also due to historical author Ted Belue and outdoor writers John Phillips and Wade Bourne for their advice and counsel to a first-time author and to Gigi Dawson for her help in preparing the manuscript for final submission.

This book is dedicated to the memory of my father:

Kenneth R. "Jap" Shupe

A man among men, and the finest example of a human being that I have ever known.

INTRODUCTION

*T*he map on page 18 is the key to the expedient use of this book in making a certain identification of a snake seen or encountered in the outdoors. Though the map is loosely based on what naturalists call the physiographic provinces of the United States, the map is an arbitrary creation of the author, and the regional divisions do not necessarily represent the true physiographic regions of the country. I have taken the liberty of creating the regional divisions shown on the map for the purposes of this book only, in an attempt to make it less cumbersome to use. It is important to note that wild animals in general and snakes in particular do not recognize political boundaries or lines drawn on a map. The actual ranges of wild animals are much more closely related to geography than to state boundary lines. Thus, to designate regions using state boundary lines alone would greatly increase the difficulty of using this book for its intended purpose, which is to quickly and accurately determine whether or not a particular snake is a dangerous, venomous species.

To help the reader more easily recognize the region of the country where he of she has seen or encountered a snake, the regional divisions are superimposed over a map of the United States showing state boundary lines. With a basic understanding of where the reader is located within a given state, the reader can readily determine in which designated region he or she is located, then refer to the pages of the book showing the photographs of the dangerous snakes found within that region. For instance, the location of my home is in far western Kentucky. Referring to the map, I will see that I am located in the region designated as the Southeast Region. Turning to the page number under the map indicated for that region, I will find a series of photographs depicting the dangerous snakes of that region. Within the photo caption under each venomous snake illustrated are directions to photos of harmless snakes that may be confused with that venomous species. Careful examination of the photographs will hopefully determine the identity of the snake.

The captions provided for each photograph also identify the snake, giving both the common name and the scientific name, as well as additional information that will help the reader distinguish the specimen from other similar snakes. In some instances where a great deal of variation exists within a species, more than one photograph of the same species may be used to aid in positive identification. For instance, Timber Rattlesnakes found within the Northeast Region regularly occur in two distinct color phases; in such a case, both color phases would be shown. Please note that even within the same species or subspecies, individual variation does occur. In fact, no two Timber Rattlesnakes will look exactly alike, just as no two horses or for that matter no two people look exactly alike. However, there are always many identifying characters that will distinguish each and every species (or subspecies).

Part of the goal of this book will be to point out to the reader those distinguishing features.

USE OF THE MAPS

*T*he most important feature in this book is the map found at the beginning of Part 2—"Using This Book to Identify a Venomous Snake."

This map, found here and on page 18, is titled "Venomous Snake Regions of the United States" and was created by the author solely for this book with the intended purpose of making venomous snake identification easier for those not

immediately eliminate all other species not found within the reader's locality, thus disposing of a great deal of confusing information that is not immediately relevant. It should be noted that there still exists the problem of the reader who finds himself located in a place on the map that is on the line of division between two or more regions. In such a case, common sense dictates that the

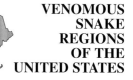

**VENOMOUS
SNAKE
REGIONS
OF THE
UNITED STATES**

SOUTHEAST REGION
NORTHEAST REGION
MIDWEST REGION
GREAT PLAINS REGION
SOUTHWEST DESERT REGION
ROCKY MOUNTAIN REGION
GREAT BASIN REGION
WEST COAST REGION

familiar with snakes. The various "venomous snake regions" created for this map are superimposed over a state map of the entire United States. After looking at the map and determining in which venomous snake region the reader is located, the reader can turn to the section of the book containing photographs of the venomous snakes of that region only. In this way it is possible to

reader should avail himself of the information provided for both regions.

The other maps found in Part 3 accompany the written information associated with the various species and subspecies and show the reader where that particular species (or subspecies) is found in the United States. As has been mentioned in the previous paragraph, some confusion may still result if the reader's locality falls on or very near the line that divides the range of one or more subspecies. Again, the reader's solution is to avail himself of the information provided for all those subspecies whose ranges are contiguous with the reader's locality.

Finally, one other confusing issue of which the reader should remain aware is the fact that the characteristics that define a population of animals as a subspecies most often change gradually rather than abruptly. Thus, a snake seen on or near the line of division between the ranges of two subspecies will probably exhibit characters common to both subspecies. In other words, it will have the appearance of being a "cross" between the two subspecies. This condition is known to biologists as "intergradation," and it is a very common occurrence among snakes. For example, if the reader's locality on the range map places them on or near the line of division between the range of the Northern Copperhead and the Southern Copperhead, a copperhead from this locale may exhibit characteristics of either the northern or southern race; or, most likely, both. The result is that a copperhead from such a locality, while still readily identifiable as a copperhead, will look more like a "cross" or "intergrade" between the northern and southern subspecies, rather than being exactly like one or the other.

EXPLANATION OF THE TEXT SECTION—(PART 3)

*F*or the benefit of those readers who wish to obtain more detailed information beyond just identifying a given snake, there is a written text section (Part 3) in this book that provides natural history information on all of America's venomous snakes.

At the end of each photo caption (Part 2) will be listed the page upon which the written information for that snake can be found. In this section the reader will be provided with a description of the natural history of the snake, as well as the author's personal observations and experiences regarding that species (or subspecies). In instances where the snake identified is represented by more than one subspecies, the written text will begin with information that is common to all subspecies, while the subsequent pages will provide information specific to each individual subspecies.

INDIVIDUAL RANGE MAPS

In the text section where natural history information is provided on each species and subspecies of a venomous snake, a range map is also provided that shows the approximate range in the United States of the snake under discussion. Taking note of these individual range maps is a valuable tool in identifying a snake. If you think the snake you saw was a copperhead, but the range map shows that copperheads are not found within your area, the odds are good that the snake you saw was not a copperhead. It should be noted that the range maps are close approximations only, but still are a useful way to quickly eliminate many snakes that are not found within the reader's area.

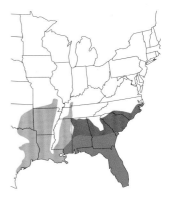

EXPLANATION OF THE USE OF SCIENTIFIC NAMES

*F*or those readers not familiar with scientific names or the concept of species and subspecies, the following explanation is provided.

Scientific names are based on the ancient languages of Latin or Greek, which makes them sound foreign to the average person with little or no background in biology. The purpose of scientific names is to avoid confusion among scientists around the world. The name "Timber Rattlesnake" in English, when translated into German or Spanish, may mean something quite different. But the scientific name of the Timber Rattlesnake, Crotalus horridus, is universal and used worldwide. Thus a Japanese scientist communicating with a German scientist would use the scientific name and both will know which animal is being discussed. This method of naming organisms can be useful even when communicating with individuals who speak the same language, since some animals may be called by different common names in different areas of the country. For instance, the snake known as a cottonmouth in Kentucky may be called water moccasin in Alabama.

Every species of animal and plant known to science has been assigned a scientific name that has two parts. The

NOTE: *Throughout this book the terms race and sub-species are used interchangeably.*

first name tells scientists the genus of the organism. The genus is a grouping of related species. Both timber rattlesnakes and eastern diamondback rattlesnakes belong to the genus Crotalus, which means that they are related species. The second name, or species name, is specific to that individual animal. Only one type of rattlesnake belonging to the genus Crotalus will have the species name horridus. In many cases, as in this book, a third scientific name is often employed. This third name refers to a subspecies of a given species. For example, the Timber Rattlesnake occurs in two distinct geographic forms, a northern mountain subspecies known as subspecies horridus (the full scientific name being written as Crotalus horridus horridus) and a southern lowland race or subspecies known as the canebrake rattlesnake, subspecies atricaudatus, with the full scientific name being written as (Crotalus horridus atricaudatus). Whenever the reader sees a scientific name with three parts, the reader will know that there is more than one geographic form of that particular snake. If only a two part scientific name is given, as in the case of the eastern diamondback rattlesnake (Crotalus adamanteus), the reader will know that there is only one geographic form of that particular animal.

The author is well aware that individuals lacking a background in biology may find this explanation of the concept of species and subspecies confusing, and thus offers the following analogy that all laymen can relate to and understand. The domestic dog goes by the sci-entific name *Canis familiaris, Canis* being the genus name. Wolves and Coyotes, which are obviously closely related to dogs, are thus also placed in the genus *canis,* but each is a different species. The wolf is *Canis lupus,* and the coyote *Canis latrans.* Thus, the dog, the wolf, and the coyote are all different species, but still closely related enough to belong to the same genus. The term subspecies is used to denote a grouping of related species. For example, German shepherds and beagles are both members of species *familiaris.* But they are obviously two different kinds of dogs, and if they were wild animals, they would be recognized as two different subspecies of the species *familiaris.* Since the differences in dogs is man made through selective breeding, science avoids using the term subspecies for different types of dogs, and instead employs the term "breed" to distinguish the different forms of domestic dog. Many scientists I know will likely cringe at this explanation of scientific nomenclature (the science of naming organisms), but the goal here is to help the lay person understand the concept of species and sub-species.

---

* In recent years the new science of DNA sequencing has resulted in many changes in the classification of America's snake species. Since the original publication of this book in 2005, the concept of subspecies has been abandoned by many herpetologists. Thus, the classifcation of snakes in this volume is somewhat different from what is seen in newer, more recently published field guides.

SOME COMMENTS ON
SNAKEBITE

*F*irst and foremost, let me state unequivocally that adequate treatment for snakebite is available only at a medical facility. The various "first-aid" measures extolled over the years (cut and suck, pack in ice, ligatures, etc.) have been proven to be largely ineffective to counterproductive and sometimes downright dangerous. Among the advice given in the arena of first aid for snakebite today are such catch 22s as "keep the victim immobilized," and "get to a hospital as soon as possible."

Such advice never seems to address the dilemma of the person alone or in a small group in the outdoors far from a hospital. How a turkey hunter bitten a half-mile from his truck located 20 miles from the nearest hospital can get there "as soon as possible" while "remaining immobilized" is never discussed in advice on snakebite first aid.

Don't despair! There is much good news about snakebite in the United States, beginning with the fact that most individuals bitten are less than an hour from the nearest hospital. Once at the hospital, a very effective therapy for snakebite exists, and fewer than three people out of a hundred bitten will die from the bite of a venomous snake in the

United States. The antivenin used to treat snakebite is highly effective in neutralizing the venom, and recent developments in the manufacture of antivenin promise to make it even more therapeutic. The author estimates as many as 75 percent of snakebites would not prove fatal even without treatment due to the fact that very often only a small amount of venom and sometimes none at all is injected by the snake. Snake venom evolved primarily as a means of securing the snake's food, and most snakes striking in defense will not inject a large amount of venom. The worst snakebites usually happen to those who work with snakes in captivity and are bitten while attempting to feed the snake. When feeding, the snake will inject a maximum amount of venom in order to kill the prey quickly before it can escape. The other type of serious snakebite usually involves a highly agitated snake that is either being handled or beaten over the head with a stick. All snakebite experts agree that the best way to get bitten in the outdoors (and, in fact the way most bites occur) is in the attempt to kill or capture the offending snake.

I have spent countless hours in the outdoors, much of them in remote

> *"...75 percent of snakebites would not prove fatal even without treatment due to the fact that very often only a small amount of venom and sometimes none at all is injected by the snake."*

wilderness, actively looking for venomous snakes, and have never been bitten by a venomous snake in the wild. Though I have been bitten more than once, every bite occurred while working in a venom production laboratory or while involved in the routine maintenance of snakes in captivity. Snakes in the wild are typically very peaceful, reclusive animals that loathe a fight. In my experience I can honestly say that the average person who enjoys the outdoors should be more concerned about being killed by a dead snag or a bolt of lightning! Still, if a giant, two-legged monster like a human comes stomping up on a snake, and the snake sees no immediate way to withdraw or remain hidden, it might bite. And if it does bite, it might inject a lethal dose of venom, and if it does that, you might die!

For those with more than a passing interest in snakebite and snake venoms, I recommend as additional reading Snakes of North America by Alan Tennant and R.D. Bartlett. The section on venoms and snakebite is very thorough and well written and though it does contain some technical terminology it is still quite informative and readable, even for those with little or no background in biology or medicine.

WHAT TO DO IF YOU SEE
A SNAKE IN THE OUTDOORS

*T*his is one of the most common questions asked of reptile experts by lay people, and the answer is exceedingly simple. Get away from it and leave it alone. For the hunter, backpacker, fisherman, hiker, etc., this is sound advice. It is of course, a different matter when the snake shows up in your backyard. Unless you (and your family) are hardcore nature lovers, it is unlikely that you want a venomous snake sharing your living area, and this would be unwise, exceptionally so if small children are involved. Children can and should be educated about snakes but, because of their natural curiosity and lack of awareness of danger, small children are often exceptionally vulnerable to snakebite, and once bitten their tiny bodies are too often unable to fight off the ravages of venom. In such a case, I reluctantly agree that a venomous snake cannot be allowed to share one's living space and for most people the safest way to dispose of it is to kill it. Don't kill harmless snakes! Their presence is very often a deterrent to the presence of dangerous species. Many harmless snakes will compete with venomous snakes for food and territory, and several, like the wide-spread kingsnakes, will regularly kill and eat venomous snakes. Members of the harmless racer clan are all confirmed eaters of venomous snakes and their young.

The safest way to kill a venomous snake if you don't have a gun is to use a long handle weapon like a garden hoe. In fact, if I were given the task of designing a primitive tool for killing snakes, I couldn't come up with a better utensil. Countless millions of snakes have likely been killed with this instrument over the years. Sadly, most were undoubtedly harmless and useful species. It should be noted that the severed head of a snake can still bite and inject a lethal dose of venom for quite some time after being removed from the body. Thus, extreme caution is advised in disposing of a recently dispatched venomous snake.

Many of my fellow reptile enthusiasts will no doubt howl with disgust on reading my instructions on how to kill a venomous snake. While I share their concerns regarding the shrinking ranges and rapid disappearance of many American snake species, I am gravely concerned about the threat these animals can pose to toddlers and small children and feel that the advice given above is the only morally responsible approach.

If, however, you encounter a snake in the wilderness, on state park or federally owned land, or even while hiking through some out-of-the-way woodland or field, you are no longer in your backyard, but in the backyard of the wild things that make this earth such a fascinating, miraculous place to live. Even dangerous snakes have the right to exist in places, and like all living things, play a roll in a scheme so grand it is beyond our ability to fathom.

PIT VIPERS AND CORAL SNAKES

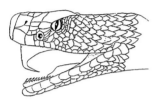

VENOMOUS
Elliptical pupil and pit

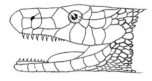

NON-VENOMOUS
Round pupil

*A*merica's venomous snakes are divided into two main groups. The largest group, known as the pit vipers, includes rattlesnakes, cottonmouths, and copperheads. Pit vipers are easily recognized by their elliptical pupils and the presence of a heat-sensory "pit" located on the side of the face between the eye and the nostril. The pit is a heat-sensitive organ that permits the snake to detect the body heat of warm-blooded prey, allowing it to strike accurately at night or in the darkness of an underground burrow. The drawing and photo clearly show the characteristics that identify a snake as a member of the pit viper group. It should be noted that while the presence of the pit and an elliptical pupil are foolproof indicators of the fact that a snake is venomous, the use of this method on a live snake in the field involves some risk. Often, getting

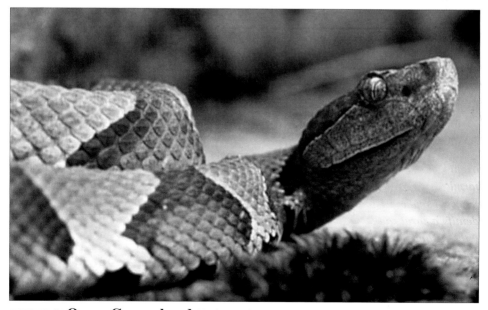

PHOTO #1 **Osage Copperhead** *(Agkistrodon contortrix phaeogaster)*
This closeup of the head of the osage copperhead clearly shows both the pit and the elliptical pupil, which are characteristics of all pit vipers.

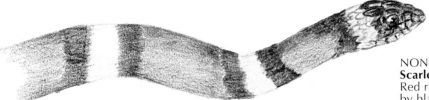

NON-VENOMOUS
Scarlet Kingsnake
Red rings bordered
by black

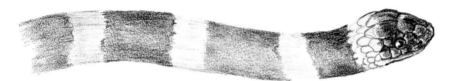

VENOMOUS
Eastern Coral Snake
Red rings bordered
by yellow

close enough to see these identifying characters means being close enough to get bitten! The drawings and photograph are useful in identifying pit vipers only. Not all venomous snakes in the United States are pit vipers!

Our other group of venomous snakes, the coral snakes, lack the pit and also have round pupils. Coral snakes are identified by color and pattern. The red, yellow, and black rings of coral snakes are distinctive, readily observed characteristics. However, not all snakes with these bright colors are venomous. Several harmless snake species closely resemble the coral snakes in color and pattern. To identify a coral snake, pay close attention to the arrangement of the colors. On all coral snakes, the red rings are bordered by yellow, while on the harmless mimics, the red rings are bordered by black. The

following poem is designed to help remember this color sequence.

"Red touches yellow,
kill a fellow,
red touches black,
venom lack."

Note on the drawing of the venomous snake the presence of the heat-sensory pit and the elliptical shape of the pupil, and on the non-venomous snake the absence of a pit and the round pupil. Photo #1 on the opposite page should give the reader an idea of how this appears on a live snake. Remember, these characters relate to pit vipers only (rattlesnakes, copperheads, cottonmouths); the dangerously venomous coral snakes lack the pit and have round pupils.

USING THIS BOOK
TO IDENTIFY
A VENOMOUS SNAKE

The first step in identifying a venomous snake using this book is to refer to the color-coded map on this page and determine in which area of the country you are located. Then use the four steps outlined below. After determining the Venomous Snake Region in which you are located, simply turn to the page(s) of photos of venomous snakes of that region and compare the photos to the snake you have seen. All venomous snakes commonly found within that region will be illustrated.

IDENTIFYING VENOMOUS SNAKES

FIRST — Look at the map on this page and determine in which region of the country you are located.

SECOND — Then locate the page number for your region, and turn to that page.

THIRD — Compare the photographs of all the venomous snakes of your region to the snake in question. You should also look at the photos of any harmless, non-venomous snakes that may be confused with a venomous species.

FOURTH — After determining the identity of the snake in question using the photo

VENOMOUS SNAKE REGIONS
OF THE UNITED STATES

graphs, note the page number for the written text section dealing with that species (or subspecies), and turn to that page for detailed written information about the snake you have identified. Also refer to the range map for that species or subspecies to be certain it occurs in your area.

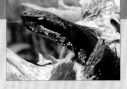

VENOMOUS
SNAKES
OF THE

SOUTHEAST
REGION

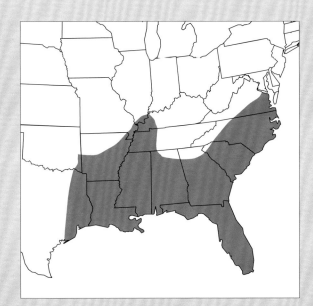

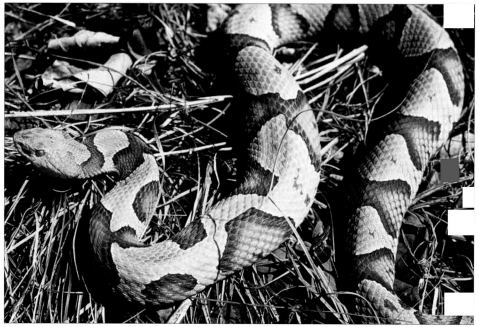

PHOTO #2 **Southern Copperhead** *(Agkistrodon contortrix contortrix)*
Note the "coppery"color of the head and the presence of darker hourglass-shaped bands across the back which are readily distinguishable characters on all copperheads. For non-venomous look-alike species see photos 66, 67, 68, and 69. Text on pages 88-89. (see also photo #3 below).

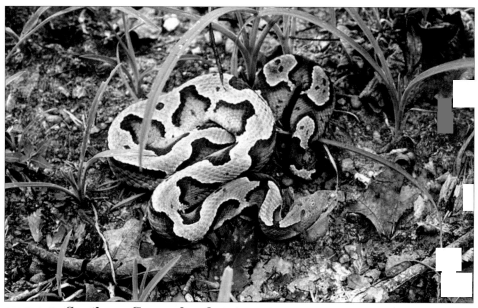

PHOTO #3 **Southern Copperhead** *(Agkistrodon contortrix contortrix)*
Note that this specimen is much browner and less coppery than the specimen shown above, a good example of the individual variation that can occur. Also notice how the dark hourglass shaped bands across the back fail to meet at the top on this specimen, a condition that is not uncommon in the Southern Copperhead and is one of the characters that separates it from all other subspecies of the copperhead (see also photo #2 above).

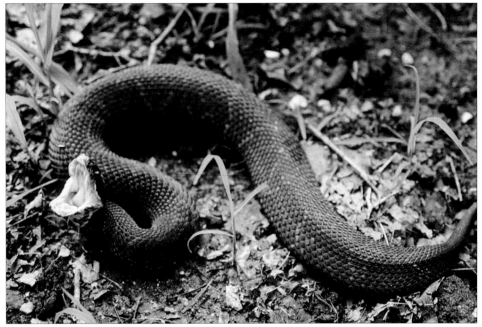

PHOTO #4 **Western Cottonmouth** *(Agkistrodon piscivorous leucostoma)*
This specimen is showing the open mouth "threat display" which has earned this species its name. An overall dark coloration is common among old adults of this species, and this western subspecies is the darkest of the three types of cottonmouths. For non-venomous look-alikes, see photos 70, 71, and 72. Text on pages 95-97 (see also photo #27).

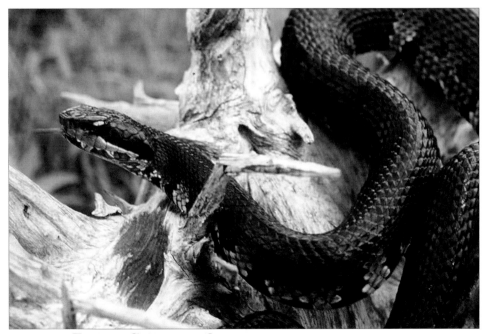

PHOTO #5 **Eastern Cottonmouth** *(Agkistrodon piscivorous piscivorous)*
Though very similar to the western subspecies shown above, Eastern Cottonmouths tend to be lighter in color and usually show some evidence of a banded pattern. For non-venomous look-alikes, see photos 73, 74, and 75. Text on page 97.

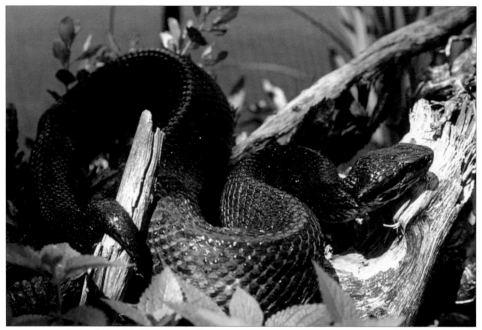

PHOTO #6 **Florida Cottonmouth** (*Agkistrodon piscivorous conanti*)
This subspecies is almost indistinguishable from the eastern form and can be told apart only by close examination of the markings on the face. Some individuals like the one shown here are quite dark, while others may exhibit the much lighter pattern common in the eastern subspecies. For non-venomous look alikes see photos 72, 74, 75, and 76. Text on pages 97-98 (*see also photo #7 below*).

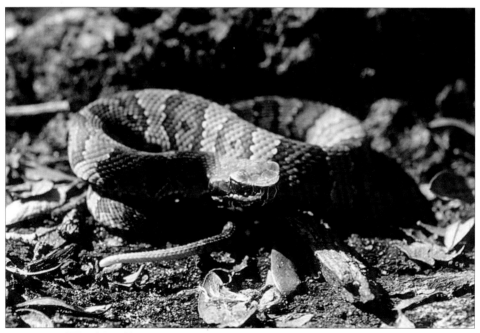

PHOTO #7 **Florida Cottonmouth** (*Agkistrodon piscivorous conanti*)
(*Young*) *Young cottonmouths of all three subspecies have a distinct banded pattern which slowly fades with age* (*see also photo #6 above*).

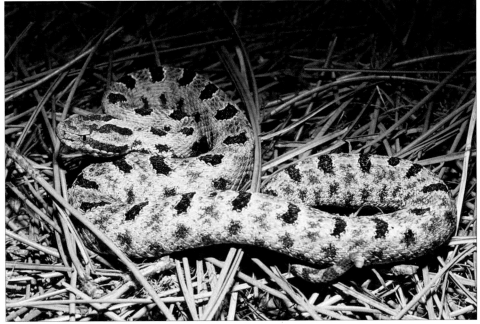

PHOTO #8 **Carolina Pygmy Rattlesnake** *(Sistrurus miliarius miliarius)*
(gray color phase) **This subspecies is highly variable in color** *(see also photo #9 below).* **For harmless look-alike, see photo #78. Text on page 100.**

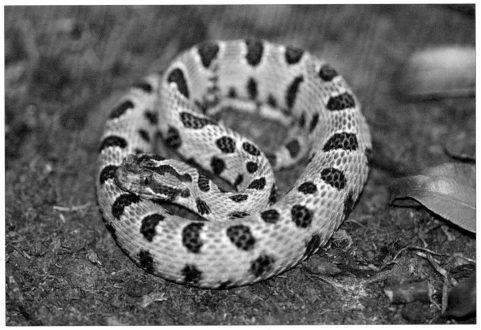

PHOTO #9 **Carolina Pygmy Rattlesnake** *(Sistrurus miliarius miliarius)*
(red color phase) **This rare color phase occurs only in the vicinity of Pamlico Sound in coastal North Carolina. Harmless look-alike species are photos 77 and 78** *(see also photo #8 above).*

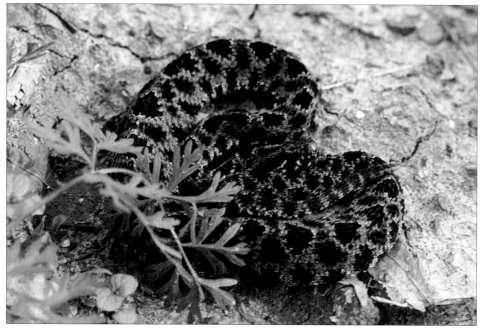

PHOTO #10 **Dusky Pygmy Rattlesnake** *(Sistrurus miliarius barbouri)*
This is the darkest and most southerly form of the three subspecies of pygmy rattlers.
Text on page 101.

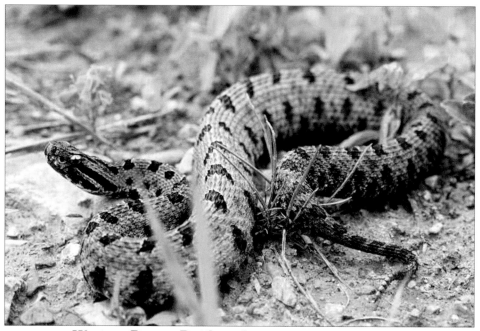

PHOTO #11 **Western Pygmy Rattlesnake** *(Sistrurus miliarius streckeri)*
(see also photo #29.) This race is much browner in color than its cousins pictured in photos 8, 9, and 10. For harmless look-alike species, see photo #78. Text on pages 101-102..

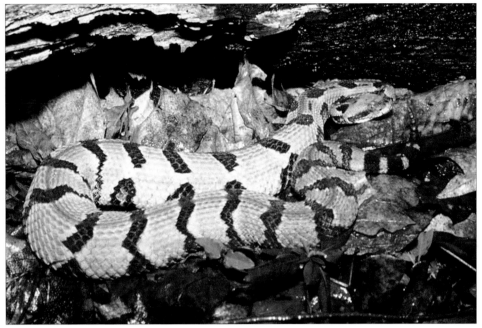

PHOTO #12 **Canebrake Rattlesnake** *(Crotalus horridus atricaudatus)*
The specimen shown in this photo is from extreme northern Florida. Compare with the specimen shown in photo #13 to get an idea of the variation that exists in canebrakes from other areas of the Southeast Region. Text on pages 111-112.

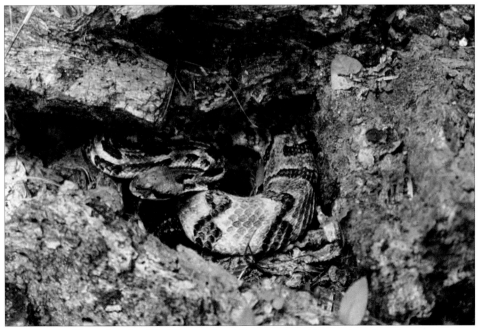

PHOTO #13 **Canebrake Rattlesnake** *(Crotalus horridus atricaudatus)*
This specimen is from western Tennessee and is typical of most canebrakes found in the Southeast Region (See also photo #12 above).

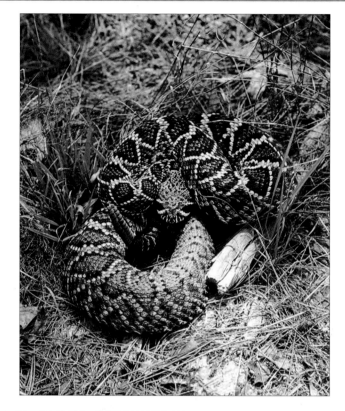

PHOTO #14
Eastern Diamondback Rattlesnake
(Crotalus adamanteus)
Generally accepted as the largest of America's rattlesnakes and certainly one of the most dangerous.
(See also photos 15 & 16.)
Text on pages 113-115.

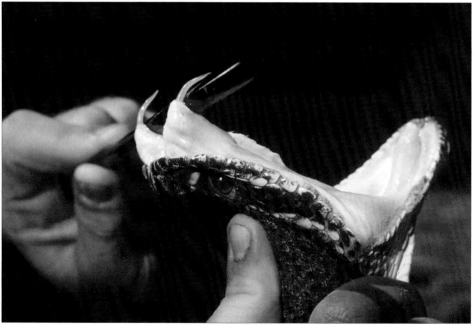

PHOTO #15 **Eastern Diamondback Rattlesnake** *(Crotalus adamanteus)*
Closeup of fangs. (See also photos 14 and 16.)

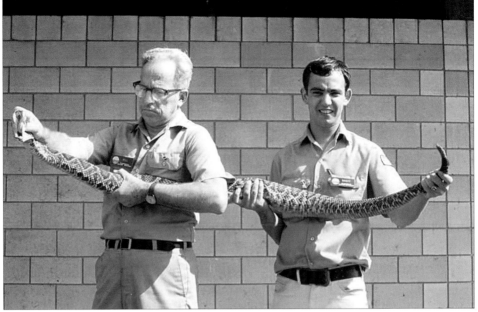

PHOTO #16 **Eastern Diamondback Rattlesnake** *(Crotalus adamanteus)*
Employees of the former Ross Allen Reptile Institute in Silver Springs, Florida show off a 6-foot 4-inch Eastern Diamondback. The year was 1971. Large individuals like this are becoming increasingly rare in the wild. A number of specimens over 7 feet have been recorded for this species, and the generally accepted record length is a whopping 8-feet 3-inches. (See also photos 14 and 15.)

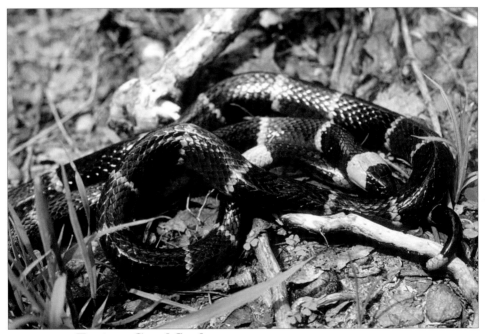

PHOTO #17 **Eastern Coral Snake** *(Micrurus fulvius fulvius)*
Coral snakes present for most people the most difficult challenge in identification. Unlike pit vipers, they have round pupils and resemble many types of harmless snakes. For non-venomous mimics, see photos 79 and 80. Text on page 148.

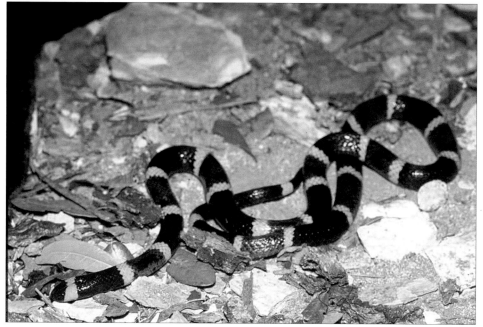

PHOTO #18 **Texas Coral Snake** *(Micrurus fulvius tenere)*
Very similar to its eastern cousin, but the Texas Coral Snake is distinguished by the large amount of black pigmentation present in the red bars. For non-venomous mimics, see photos 79 and 80. Text on page 148.

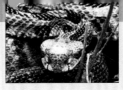

VENOMOUS
SNAKES
O F T H E

NORTHEAST
REGION

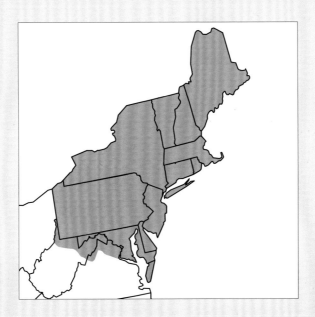

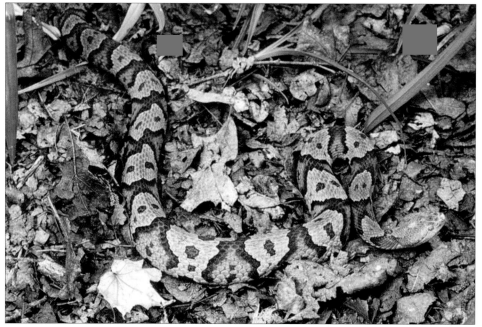

PHOTO #19 **Northern Copperhead** *(Agkistrodon contortrix mokasen)*
(See also photos 20 and 25.) **Note how well this snake's color and pattern hide it among the leaf litter. For non-venomus look-alike, see photo #81. Text on pages 86-88.**

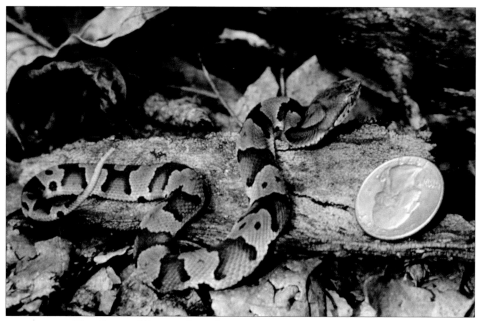

PHOTO #20 **Northern Copperhead** *(Agkistrodon contortrix contortrix)*
(Young) (See also photos 19 and 25.) **Young copperheads are miniature replicas of the adults except for the bright yellow tail tip which when wriggled resembles a grub and serves as a lure to attract lizards, invertebrates, and other small prey. The yellow tail tip fades with age. The quarter is for size reference.**

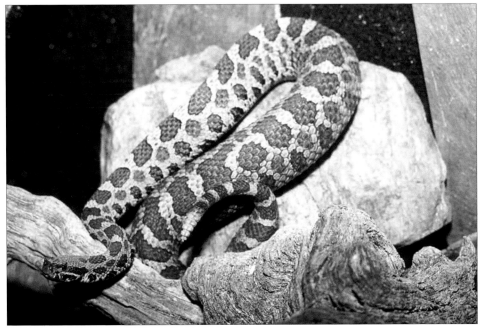

PHOTO #21 **Eastern Massasauga** *(Sistrurus catenatus catenatus)*
*(See also photo #28.) **The peculiar name of this dwarf species of rattlesnake comes from the Chippewa Indians. Text on pages 104-105.***

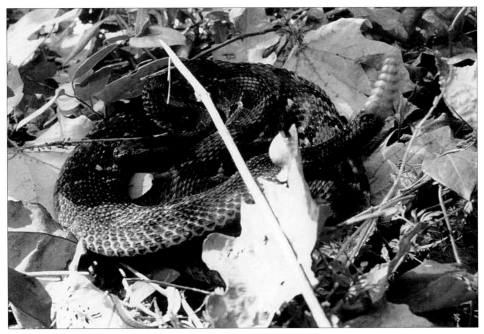

PHOTO #22 **Timber Rattlesnake** *(Crotalus horridus horridus)*
*(dark color phase) (See also photos 23, 24, and 30.) **Some dark phase individuals will be almost totally black, though most will show some evidence of a pattern. Text on pages 108-110.***

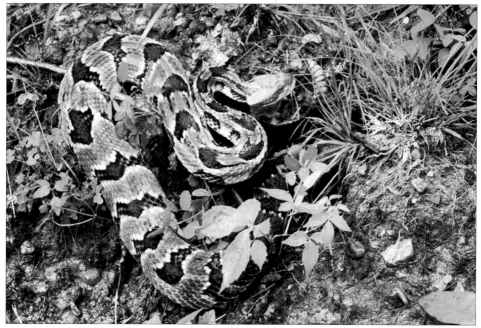

PHOTO #23 **Timber Rattlesnake** *(Crotalus horridus horridus)*
(light phase) (See also photos 22, 24, and 30.) **Some light phase individuals from the northeastern most portion of their range are sulphur yellow in coloration. Text on pages 108-110.**

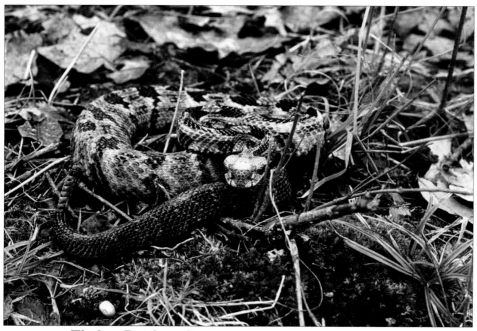

PHOTO #24 **Timber Rattlesnake** *(Crotalus horridus horridus)*
(See also photos 22, 23, and 30.) **This specimen is intermediate between the light and dark phases and is typical of specimens found throughout much of this snake's range.**

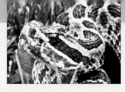

VENOMOUS
SNAKES
OF THE

MIDWEST
REGION

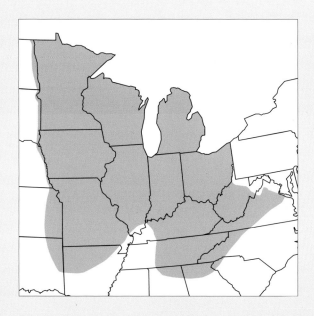

PHOTO #25
Northern Copperhead
(Agkistrodon contortrix contortrix)
*(See also photos 19 & 20) **This photo provides another good example of the copperhead's excellent camouflage when lying among dead leaves on the forest floor. For harmless look-alike species, see photos 81, 82, 83 and 84. Text on pages 86-88.***

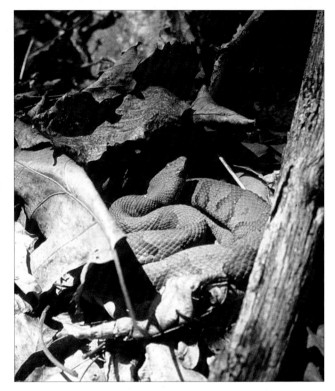

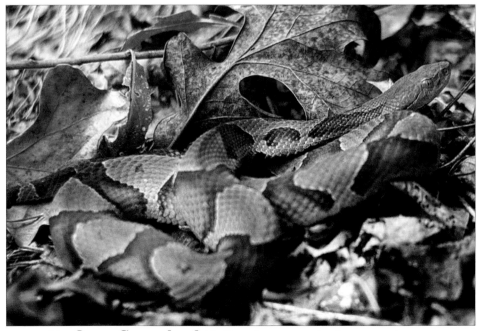

PHOTO #26 **Osage Copperhead** *(Agkistrodon contortrix phaeogaster)*
*(See also photo #1.) **This subspecies is very similar to the Southern Copperhead (photos 2 and 3), but is usually browner in color and has the dark crossbands edged in light pigment. Harmless look alike shown in photos 81, 83 and 84. Text on pages 89-90.***

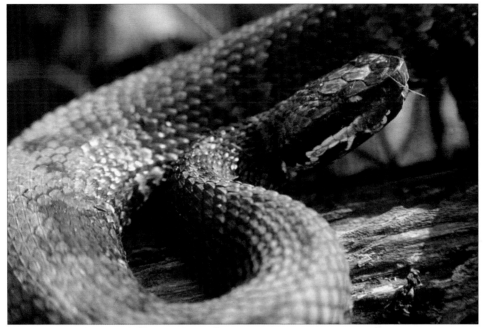

PHOTO #27 **Western Cottonmouth** *(Agkistrodon piscivorous leucostoma)*
(See also photo #4.) This is the smallest, darkest, and most northerly ranging of the three subspecies of cottonmouths in America. Confusing non-venomous species are shown in photos 70, 71 and 85. Text on pages 95-97.

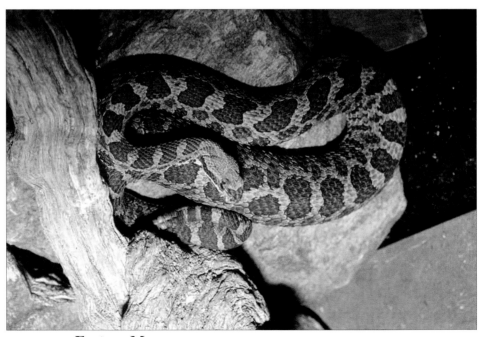

PHOTO #28 **Eastern Massasauga** *(Sistrurus catenatus catenatus)*
(See also photo #21.) Because most of this snake's range is located in the heavily farmed Corn Belt region of America, little of its original habitat remains. Today these snakes occur only in widely scattered localities where remnants of the original habitat remain. Text on pages 104-105.

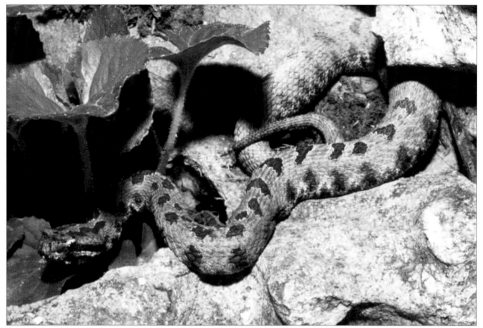

PHOTO #29 **Western Pygmy Rattlesnake** *(Sistrurus miliarius streckeri)*
(See also photo #11.) **Found in the Midwest Region only in the Ozark highlands of south-central Missouri and northwestern Arkansas. For harmless look alikes see photo #78. Text on pages 101-102.**

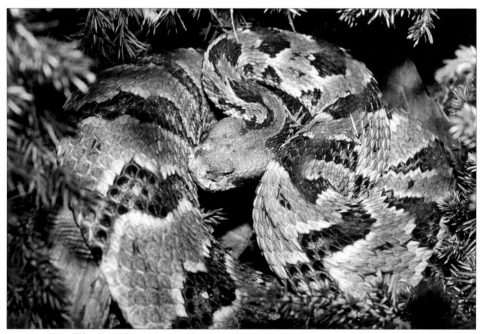

PHOTO #30 **Timber Rattlesnake** *(Crotalus horridus horridus)*
(See also photos 22, 23 and 24.) **Though widespread throughout the Midwest Region, this snake today is found only in areas of remaining habitat and is becoming increasingly rare. Text on pages 108-110.**

*T*he following snakes are species whose ranges barely enter into the Midwest Region from other regions where they may be common and widespread.

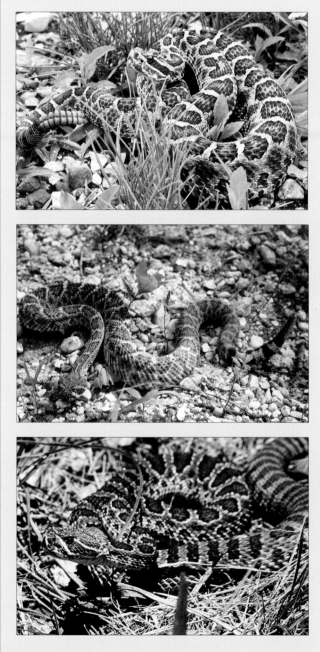

PHOTO #32
Western Massasauga
(Sistrurus catenatus tergiminus)
Found mostly in the Great Plains Region, but enters the Midwest Region in the southeastern corner of Iowa and extreme north-western Missouri.

PHOTO #34
Western Diamondback Rattlesnake
(Crotalus atrox)
Found mostly in the southern Great Plains Region and the Southwest Desert Region; it barely extends its range into the Midwest Region into west central Arkansas.

PHOTO #33
Prairie Rattlesnake
(Crotalus viridis viridis)
Commonly found in the Great Plains and Rocky Mountain Regions, its range barely extends into the Midwest Region in the "Loess Hills" area of northwestern Iowa.

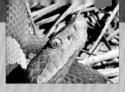

VENOMOUS
SNAKES
O F   T H E

GREAT PLAINS
REGION

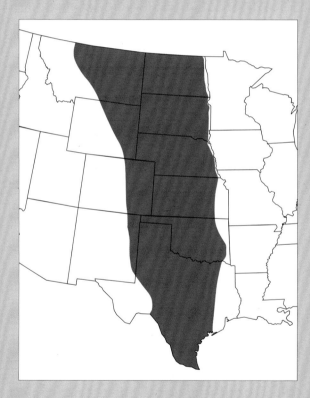

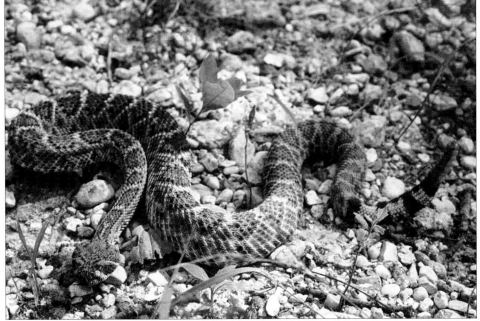

PHOTO #34 **Western Diamondback Rattlesnake** *(Crotalus atrox)*
This snake is widespread throughout the southern Great Plains Region and the Southwest Desert Region; it barely extends its range into the Midwest Region into west central Arkansas. Text on pages 116-118.

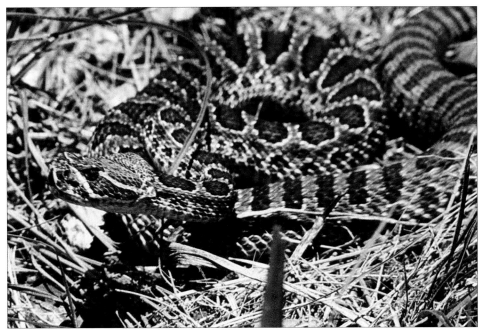

PHOTO #33 **Prairie Rattlesnake** *(Crotalus viridis viridis)*
Commonly found in the Great Plains and Rocky Mountain Regions, the Prairie Rattlesnake's range barely extends into the Midwest Region in the "Loess Hills" area of northwestern Iowa. Text on pages 120-121.

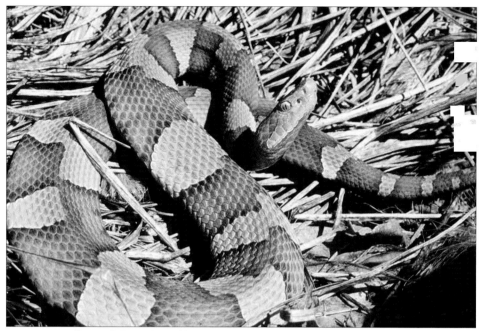

PHOTO #31 **Broad Banded Copperhead** *(Agkistrodon contortrix laticinctus)*
This subspecies differs from the Northern, Southern, and Osage Copperheads in having much wider dark bands across the back. Text on page 90.

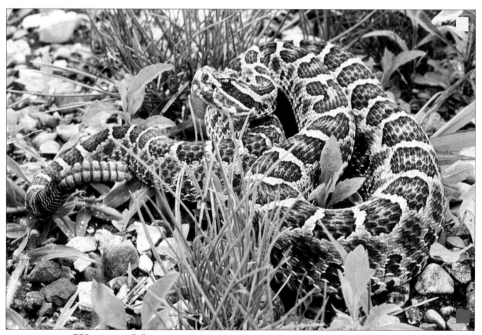

PHOTO #32 **Western Massasauga** *(Sistrurus catenatus tergiminus)*
Except for a tiny area of the Midwest Region, this snake's entire range is contained within the Great Plains Region. For harmless look-alikes, see photos 86 and 92. Text on page 105.

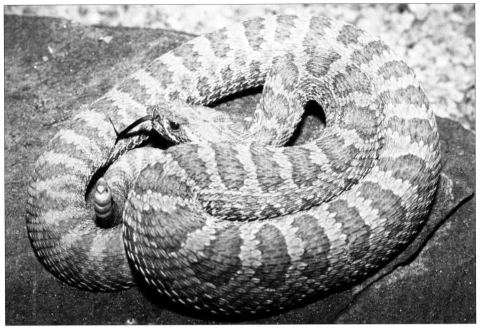

PHOTO #58 **Prairie Rattlesnake** *(Crotalus viridis viridis)*
In the Rocky Mountain Region, this rattler can be found in grasslands, canyons, and mountain slopes as high as 10,000 feet in elevation. (See also photos 55 and 33.) For harmless snakes that are sometimes confused with the Prairie rattler, see photo #87. Text on pages 120-121.

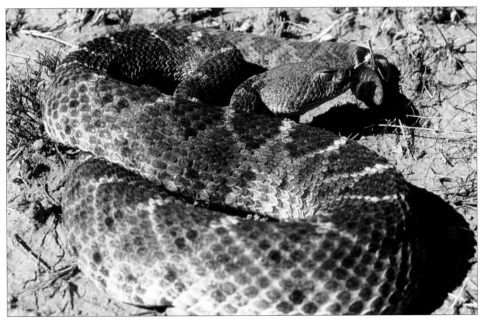

PHOTO #38 **Western Diamondback Rattlesnake** *(Crotalus atrox)*
(See also photo #34.) A large, dangerous snake with an irascible disposition, the Western Diamondback is credited with more snakebite deaths than any other North American serpent, but its venom is actually less potent than many other rattlesnakes. Text on pages 116-118.

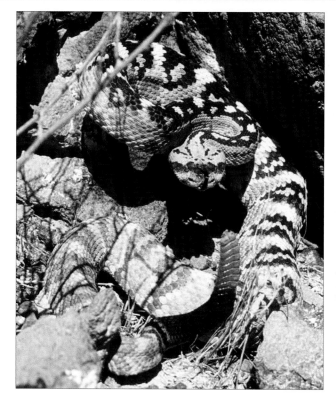

PHOTO #35

Black-Tailed Rattlesnake

(Crotalus molossus molossus)
Note the jet black tail which lends this species its name. This snake is found in the Great Plains Region in central and western Texas, as well as being widespread in much of the Southwest Desert Region. Compare this specimen from west Texas to photo #45 (an Arizona specimen) to get an idea of the geographic variation that exists in this species. Text on pages 129-180.

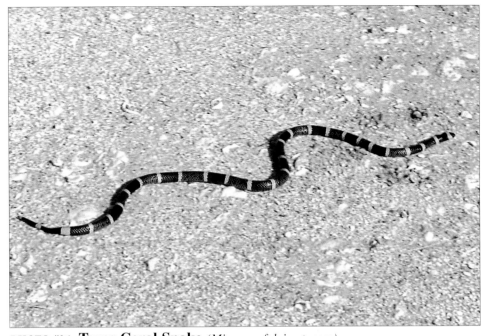

PHOTO #36 **Texas Coral Snake** *(Micrurus fulvius tenere)*
(See also photo #18.) **While also found in parts of the Southeast Region, in the Great Plains Region the Texas Coral can be found only in eastern and southern Texas. For harmless mimics, see photos 79, 80 and 88. Text on page 148.**

*T*he following are additional snake species whose ranges barely enter the Great Plains Region, but may be common and widespread in other regions.

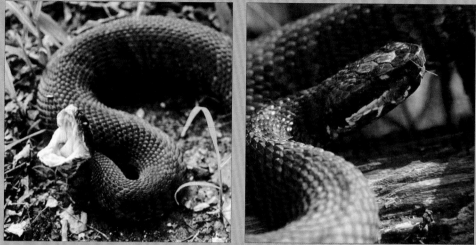

PHOTOS # 4 (ABOVE LEFT) AND # 27 (ABOVE RIGHT)
Western Cottonmouth *(Agkistrodon piscivorous leucostoma)*
In the Great Plains Region, these snakes are found in southeastern Oklahoma and parts of central Texas. Text on pages 95-97.

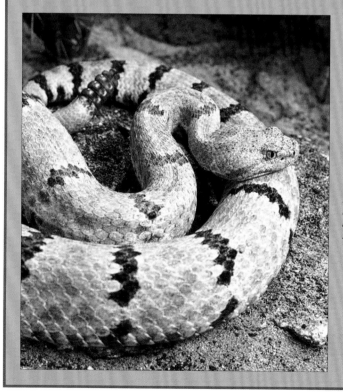

PHOTO #42
Mottled Rock Rattlesnake
(Crotalus lepidus lepidus)
Found mostly in the Southwest Desert Region, but ranging into the Great Plains Region in southwestern Texas. Text on page 132.

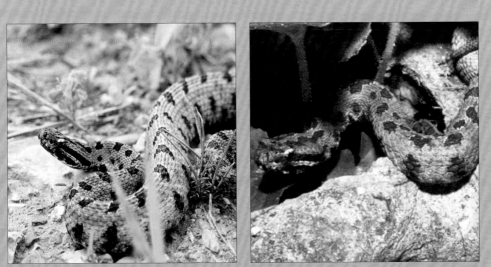

PHOTOS #11 (ABOVE LEFT) AND #29 (ABOVE RIGHT)
Western Pygmy Rattlesnake *(Sistrurus miliarius streckeri)*
This snake's range barely enters the Great Plains Region in southeastern Oklahoma and north-east Texas. Text on pages 101-102.

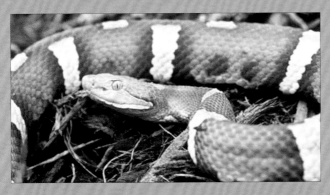

PHOTO #57
Trans-Pecos Copperhead
(Agkistrodon contortrix pictigaster)
This westernmost subspecies of the copperhead is found mostly in the Big Bend area of Texas, which is in the Southwest Desert Region. It does range into the Great Plains Region in a small area of southwestern Texas. Text on page 91.

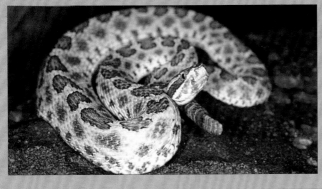

PHOTO #40
Desert Massasauga
(Sistrurus catenatus edwardsi)
A rare snake occurring in wide-ly scattered populations mostly in the Southwest Desert Region but also in the Great Plains Region in a few places in the Texas Panhandle and extreme southeastern Texas. See range map on page 103. Text on page 106.

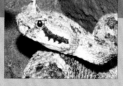

VENOMOUS
SNAKES
O F   T H E

*SOUTHWEST
DESERT
REGION*

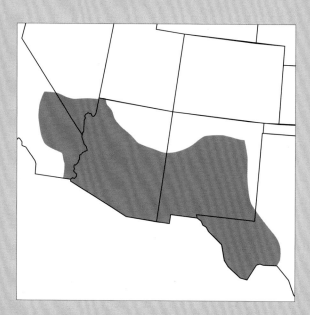

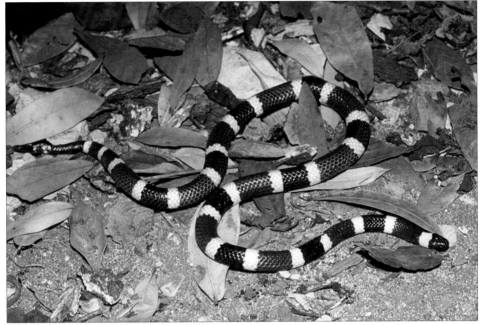

PHOTO #37 **Western Coral Snake** *(Micruroides euryxanthus)*
This snake is found mostly in Arizona, but also ranges into extreme southeastern New Mexico. These are secretive little snakes that are not often observed. For non-venomous look-alike species, see photos 88, 89 and 96. Text on page 149.

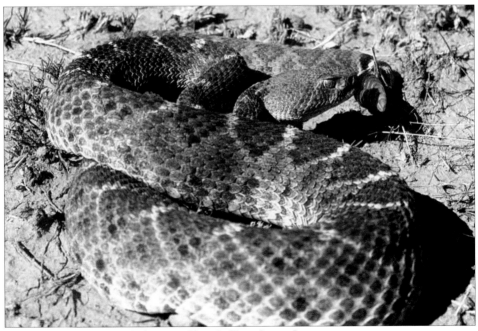

PHOTO #38 **Western Diamondback Rattlesnake** *(Crotalus atrox)*
(See also photo #34.) A large, dangerous snake with an irascible disposition, the Western Diamondback is credited with more snakebite deaths than any other North American serpent, but its venom is actually less potent than many other rattlesnakes. Text on pages 116-118.

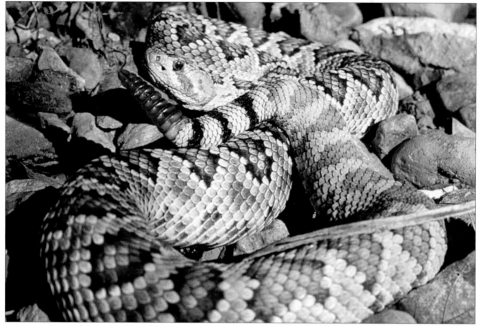

PHOTO #39 **Mojave Rattlesnake** *(Crotalus scutulatus scutulatus)*
Very similar to the Western Diamondback, but even more dangerous! Note the alternate black and white rings on the tail, a trait shared with the Western Diamondback, but on the Mojave Rattlesnake the black rings are narrower than the white rings. Text on pages 127-128.

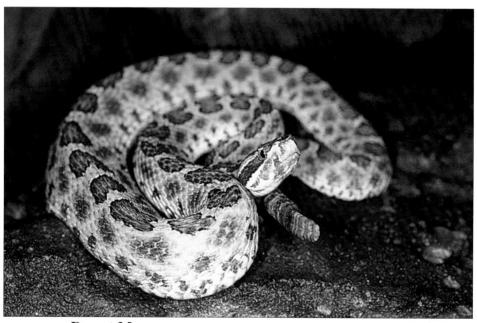

PHOTO #40 **Desert Massasauga** *(Sistrurus catenatus edwardsi)*
This rare little rattlesnake occurs mostly in desert grassland habitats. Much of its habitat has been destroyed or altered by overgrazing, and today this snake is distributed in widely disjointed locales where good habitat remains. For harmless look-alike species, see photos 86, 87 and 91. Text on page 106.

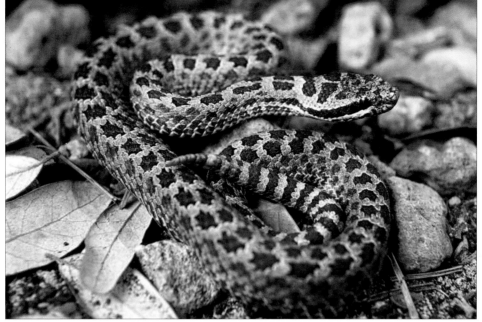

PHOTO #41 **Twin-Spotted Rattlesnake** *(Crotalus pricei pricei)*
This is a small, rare snake found only in the higher elevations of a half-dozen small, desert mountain ranges in southeastern Arizona. Most specimens show a twin row of dark spots on the back, which give the snake its name. On occasional older specimens the double row of spots may fade, leaving an almost uniformly grayish brown snake. Text on pages 133-134.

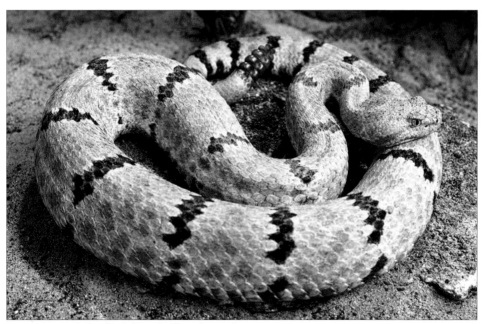

PHOTO #42 **Mottled Rock Rattlesnake** *(Crotalus lepidus lepidus)*
This snake is found only in the "Big Bend" region of Texas and southward into Mexico. Note how well the color on this specimen matches the color of the rock where it lives, a condition that is common among the Rock Rattlesnakes. For harmless snakes sometimes confused with this rattlesnake, see photo #90. Text on page 132.

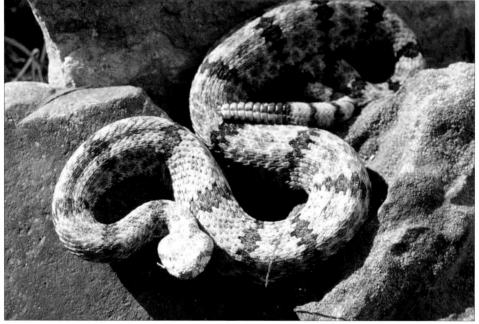

PHOTO #43 **Banded Rock Rattlesnake** *(Crotalus lepidus klauberi)*
The name "Rock Rattlesnake" is very appropriate for this small rattler as it is usually found among rocks. Their highly variable color always matches the color of the rocks where they live (see also photo #44). Text on pages 132-133.

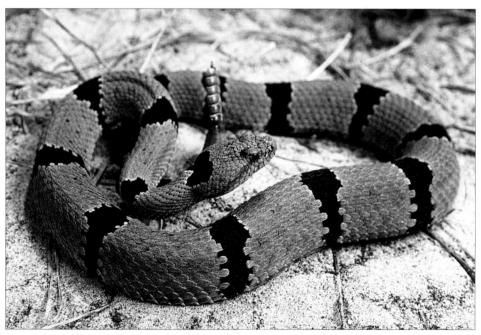

PHOTO #44 **Banded Rock Rattlesnake** *(Crotalus lepidus klauberi)*
These handsome little rattlers are highly variable in color, with their color matching the color of the rocks where they live (See also photo #43 above). For non-venomous look-alike, see photo #90. Text on pages 132-133.

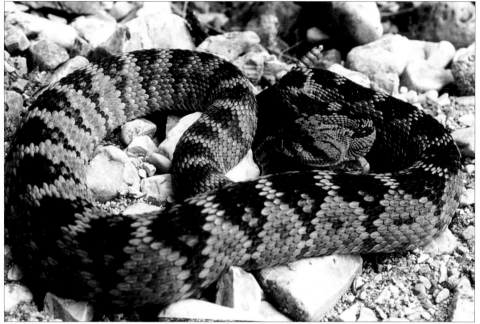

PHOTO #45 **Black-Tailed Rattlesnake** (*Crotalus molossus molossus*)
Note the jet black tail from which this snake derives its name. This species is also found in parts of the Great Plains Region in south-central Texas, but specimens from that area are different in color (see photo #35). The specimen pictured here is from Arizona and is typical of specimens from the Southwest Desert Region. Text on pages 129-130.

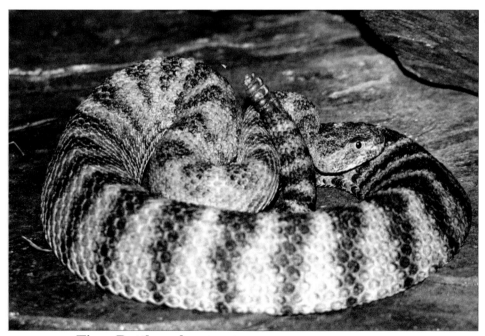

PHOTO #46 **Tiger Rattlesnake** (*Crotalus tigris*)
Note the especially small head on this rattlesnake, which many herpetologists believe is an adaptation for hunting lizards and other small prey hidden within narrow rock crevices. In the United States these snakes can be found only in south-central Arizona. Text on pages 137-138.

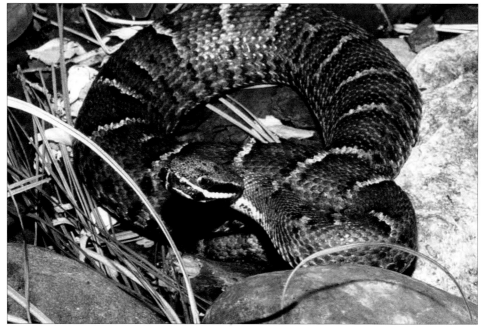

PHOTO #47 **Arizona Ridge-Nosed Rattlesnake** *(Crotalus willardi willardi)*
These small mountain rattlesnakes are very local in occurrence, being found only in three desert mountain ranges in southern Arizona: the Patagonia, Santa Rita, and Huachuca Mountains. Text on page 136.

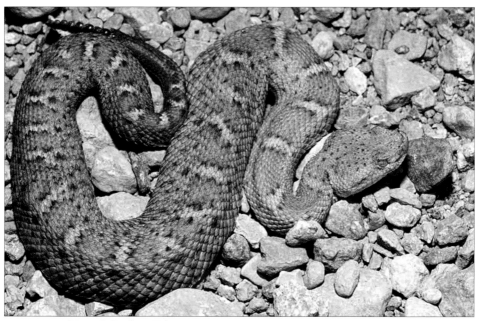

PHOTO #48 **New Mexico Ridge-Nosed Rattlesnake** *(Crotalus willardi obscurus)*
This small rattler is found in the United States in only two desert mountain ranges: the Animas Mountains and the Peloncillo Mountains of extreme southwestern New Mexico. Because of their highly restricted range, these snakes are considered a threatened species and are protected by law. Text on pages 136-137.

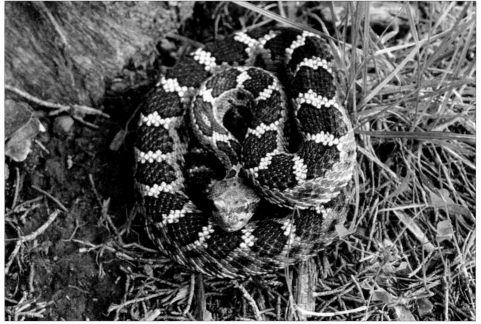

PHOTO #49 **Arizona Black Rattlesnake** *(Crotalus viridis cerberus)*
As their name implies, this is one of America's darkest rattlesnakes, and some are jet black. This is another mountain race, found in the higher elevations of the "Mogollon Rim" area of central Arizona and west-central New Mexico. Text on page 126.

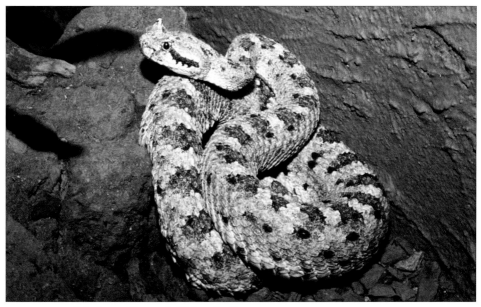

PHOTO #50 **Mojave Desert Sidewinder** *(Crotalus cerastes cerastes)*
This is one of three forms of the famed "Sidewinder Rattlesnake," whose name is derived from its unique form of locomotion. The Mojave Desert Sidewinder is the northernmost form of the three subspecies. Found mostly in the Mojave Desert, its range extends slightly into the West Coast Region and the Great Basin Region. Note the hornlike projections above the eye in all three sidewinder subspecies. Text on page 145.

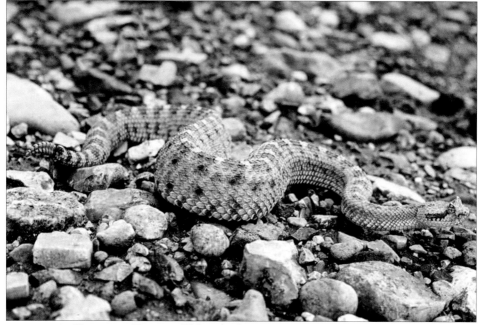

PHOTO #51 **Sonoran Desert Sidewinder** *(Crotalus cerastes cercobombus)*
As its name implies, this subspecies is found in the Sonoran Desert of south-central Arizona and northwestern Mexico. Differences among the three subspecies of sidewinders are so slight that even experts can have difficulty telling them apart unless they know the locality where they were found. Text on page 145.

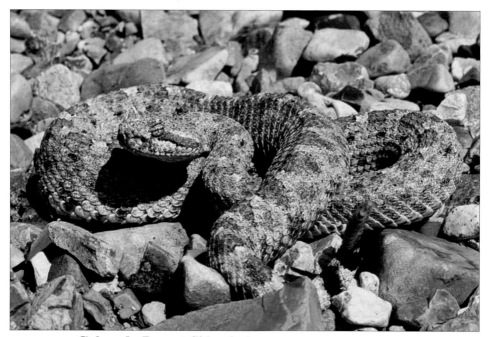

PHOTO #52 **Colorado Desert Sidewinder** *(Crotalus cerastes laterorepens)*
As its name implies, this is a snake of the Colorado desert area of southeastern California and extreme southwestern Arizona. A small portion of its range extends into the West Coast Region. Text on page 145.

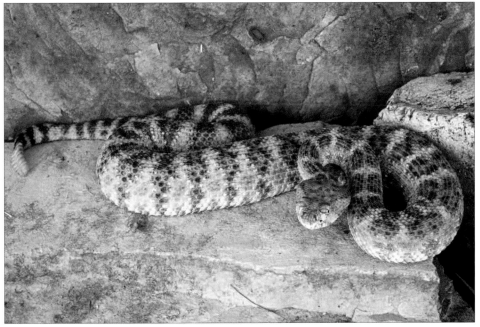

PHOTO #53 **Southwestern Speckled Rattlesnake** *(Crotalus mitchelli pyrrhus)*
This is probably the most variable colored rattlesnake in the southwestern United States, its speckled color always matching the predominant color of the rocks and gravel where it lives. (See also photo #65.) Text on pages 140-141.

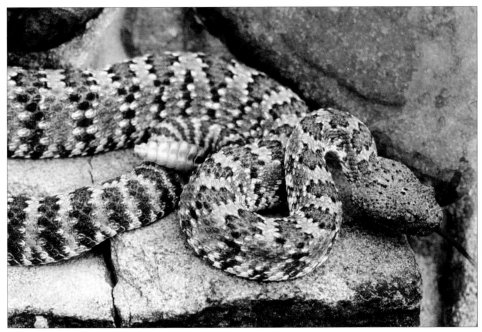

PHOTO #54 **Panamint Rattlesnake** *(Crotalus mitchelli stephensi)*
This snake inhabits some of the harshest environments in America. Its name comes from the Panamint Mountains of California's Death Valley. Text on page 140.

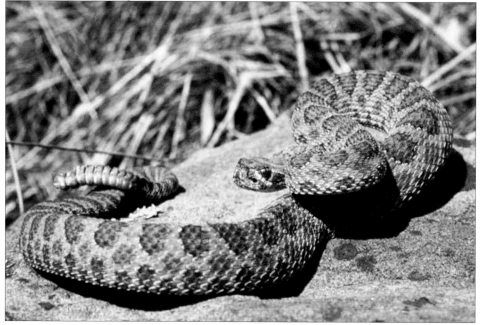

PHOTO #55 **Prairie Rattlesnake** *(Crotalus viridis viridis)*
America's most wide-spread venomous snake, the Prairie rattler is found in the Great Plains and Rocky Mountain Regions as well as portions of the Southwest Desert Region. (See also photo #33 and photo #58.) **For non-venomous look-alikes, see photos 91 and 92. Text on pages 120-121.**

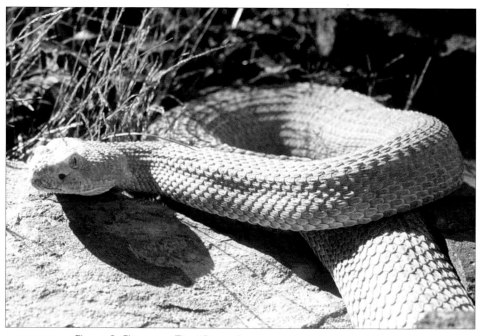

PHOTO #56 **Grand Canyon Rattlesnake** *(Crotalus viridis abyssus)*
This is one of the rarest rattlesnakes in America, being found only in the vicinity of the Grand Canyon. It is a protected species. Text on page 125.

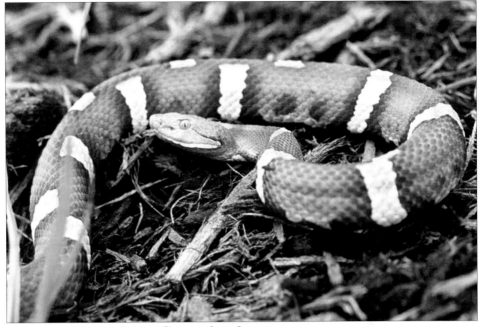

PHOTO #57 **Trans-Pecos Copperhead** *(Agkistrodon contortrix pictigaster)*
In the Southwest Desert Region, this snake can be found only in the Big Bend area of west Texas. Text on page 91.

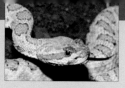

VENOMOUS
SNAKES
OF THE

ROCKY
MOUNTAIN
REGION

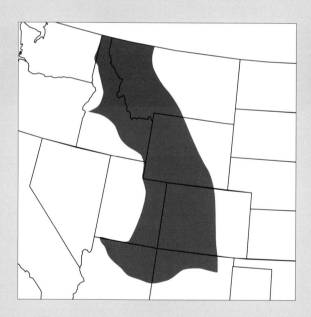

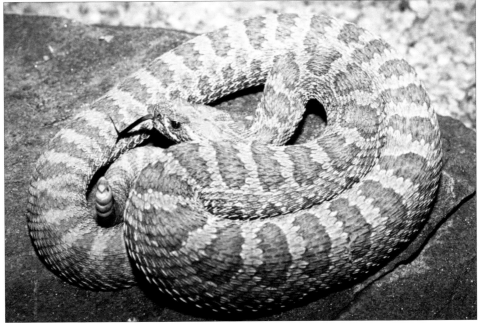

PHOTO #58 **Prairie Rattlesnake** *(Crotalus viridis viridis)*
In the Rocky Mountain Region, this rattler can be found in grasslands, canyons, and mountain slopes as high as 10,000 feet in elevation. (See also photos 55 and 33.) For harmless snakes that are sometimes confused with the Prairie rattler, see photo #87. Text on pages 120-121.

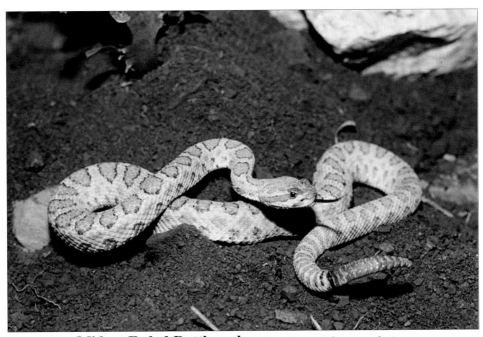

PHOTO #59 **Midget Faded Rattlesnake** *(Crotalus viridis concolor)*
This small, uncommon rattlesnake is found mostly in western Colorado and eastern Utah, as well as a small area of southwestern Wyoming. It possesses a highly toxic venom and despite its small size, bites from this snake can be very serious. Text on page 126.

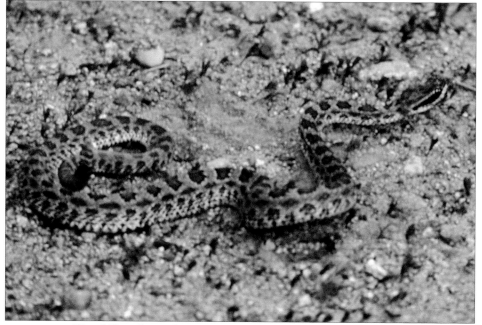

PHOTO #60 **Hopi Rattlesnake** *(Crotalus viridis nuntius)*
This is another smallish member of the Western Rattlesnake group, which includes eight sub-species of Crotalus viridis. *Its name is derived from the Hopi Indian tribe, which historically used these snakes in ceremonial dances. Very similar to the Prairie Rattlesnake. For harmless look-alike species, see photos 92 and 95. Text on page 125.*

*T*he following snake barely
enters into the Rocky
Mountain Region. Other photos
appear elsewhere.

Northern Pacific Rattlesnake
(Crotalus viridis oreganus)
(See photo #63 at right.) **Most of this
snake's range is contained in the West
Coast Region. It barely enters the Rocky
Mountain Region in north-central Idaho.**

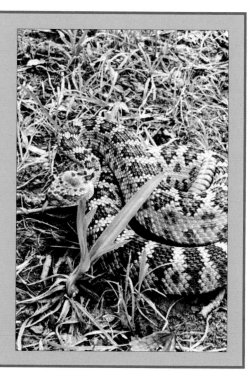

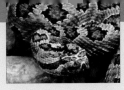

VENOMOUS
SNAKES
O F   T H E

GREAT BASIN
REGION

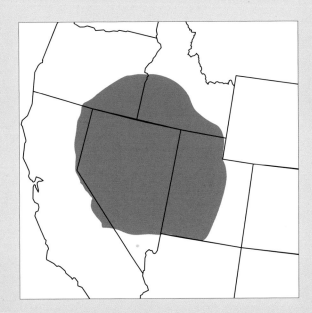

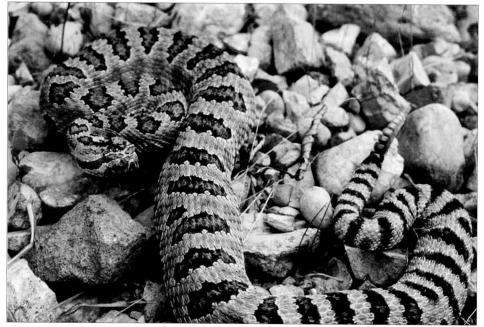

PHOTO #61 **Great Basin Rattlesnake** *(Crotalus viridis lutosus)*
This rather large rattlesnake can be found throughout the Great Basin Region. For non-venomous snakes sometimes confused with the Great Basin rattler, see photo #93. Text on page 124.

The following two snakes are species whose range barely enters into the Great Plains Region.

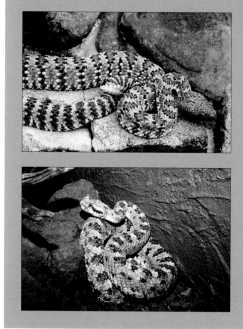

Panamint Rattlesnake

(Crotalus mitchelli stephensi)
(See photo #54 at left.) **The heart of this snake's range is in California's Death Valley in the West Coast Region; it ranges eastward into the Great Basin Region in southwestern Nevada.**

Mojave Desert Sidewinder

(Crotalus cerastes cerastes)
(See photo #50 at left.) **This snake ranges northward from the Southwest Desert Region into the Great Basin Region in southern Nevada and extreme southwestern Utah.**

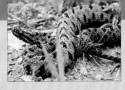

VENOMOUS
SNAKES
OF THE

WEST COAST
REGION

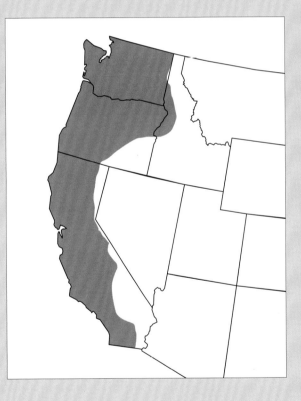

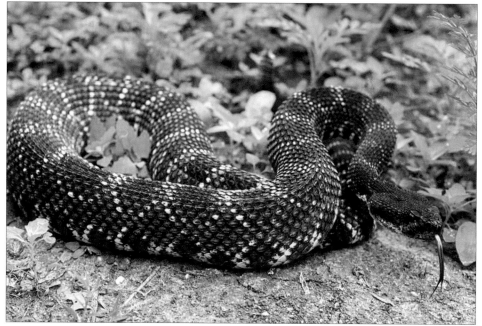

PHOTO #62 **Southern Pacific Rattlesnake** (*Crotalus viridis helleri*)
This is one of the largest members of the eight forms of the Western Rattlesnake group (*Crotalus viridis*). *It is found only in southwestern California. Text on page 123.*

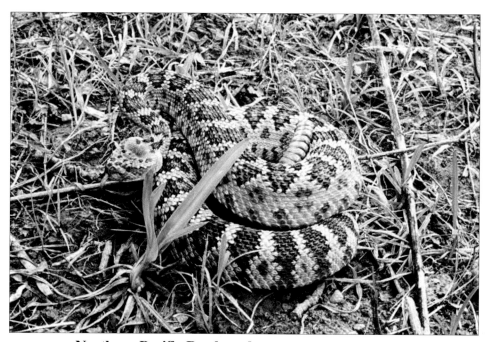

PHOTO #63 **Northern Pacific Rattlesnake** (*Crotalus viridis oreganus*)
Very similar to the Southern Pacific Rattlesnake (*photo #62 above*), *but lighter in color and having a much greater range. For non-venomous look-alike species, see photo #94. Text on page 122.*

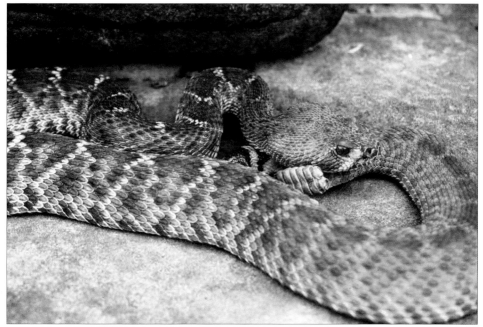

PHOTO #64 **Red Diamond Rattlesnake** *(Crotalus exsul ruber)*
These large, robust rattlers have a rather small range in the United States, being found only in a small area of Southwestern California. Like many species in the western United States however their range extends southward into Mexico. Text on pages 141-142.

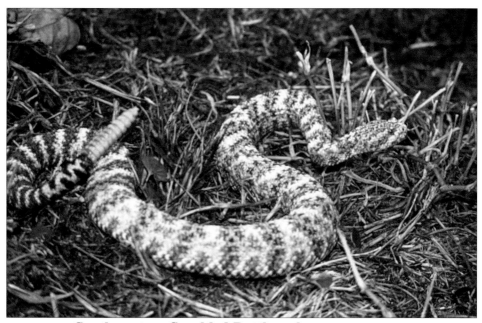

PHOTO #65 **Southwestern Speckled Rattlesnake** *(Crotalus mitchelli pyrrhus)*
This rattlesnake is extremely variable in color, with its speckled pattern often matching exactly the color of the gravel substrate where it lives. (See also photo #53.) In the West Coast Region, this snake is found only in southwestern California, being more widespread in the Southwest Desert Region. Text on pages 140-141.

*T*he following are snakes whose ranges bare-ly enter into the West Coast Region from the Southwest Desert Region.

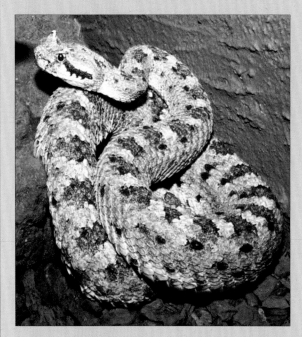

PHOTO #50
Mojave Desert Sidewinder
(Crotalus cerastes cerastes)
Found in the West Coast Region desert areas of east-central California. Text on page 145.

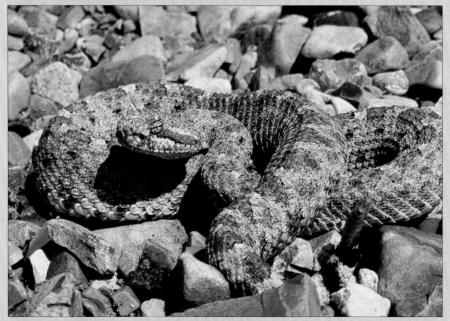

PHOTO #52 **Colorado Desert Sidewinder** *(Crotalus cerastes laterorepens)*
This snake's range barely enters the West Coast Region in extreme southwest California. Text on page 145.

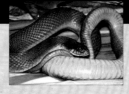

NON-VENOMOUS
MIMICS

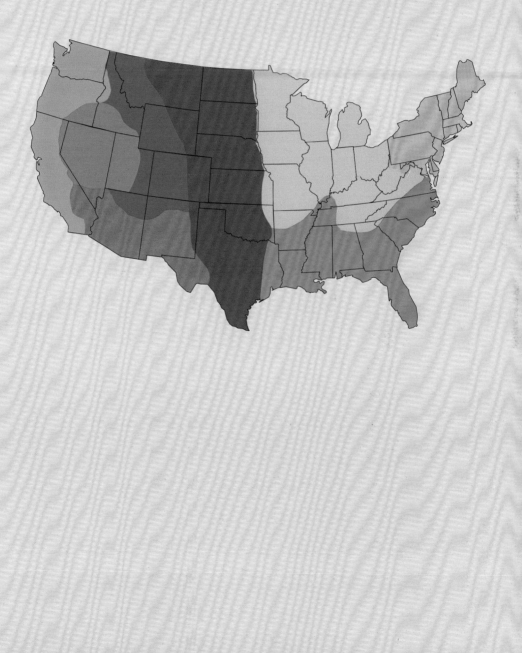

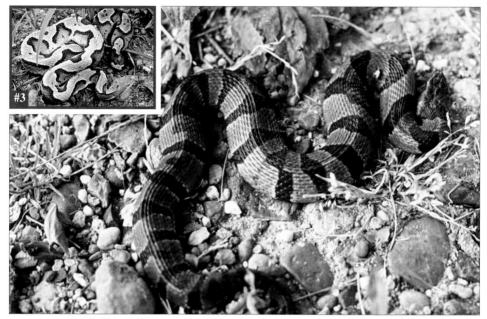

PHOTO #66 **Midland Water Snake** *(Nerodia sipedon pleuralis)*
*Because these snakes have a pattern of crossbands on the back and their color scheme is brown,
reddish, or coppery, they are often confused with the Southern Copperhead #3. Note that on the
Midland Water Snake, the dark bands are wider at the top and narrower on the sides. On the
Copperhead, the opposite is true, with the dark bands being wider on the sides and narrow on the
top. Also note round pupils and lack of facial "pit."*

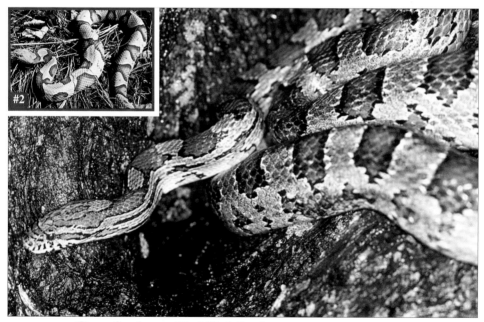

PHOTO #67 **Corn Snake or Red Rat Snake** *(Elaphe guttata guttata)*
*This snake's overall reddish coloration, especially on the head, has caused it to sometimes be
confused with the Southern Copperhead #2. Note round pupils and lack of "pit"; also note the
presence of dark blotches on the back as opposed to dark bands, all characteristics which differentiate from copperhead.*

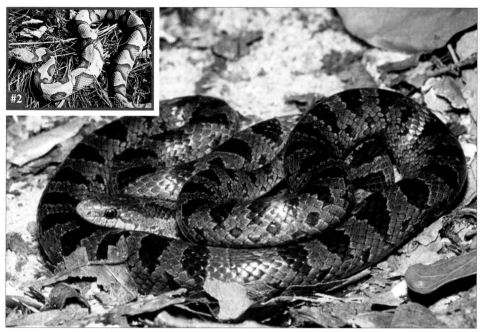

PHOTO #68 **Mole Kingsnake** *(Lampropeltis calligaster rhombomaculata)*
The russet color on the head and dorsal blotches leads to this snake sometimes being confused with the Southern Copperhead #2. Note round pupil and lack of "pit"; also note the presence of rhomboid-shaped blotches on the back as opposed to bands, all characteristics which differentiate from the Copperhead.

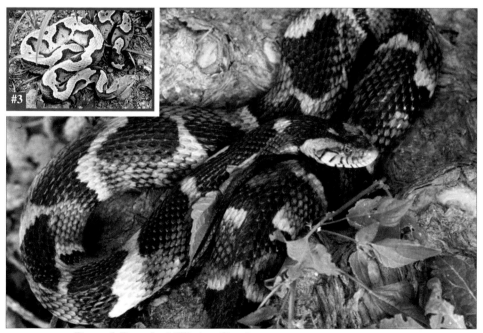

PHOTO #69 **Broad Banded Water Snake** *(Nerodia fasciata confluens)*
Sometimes confused with the Southern Copperhead #3. But despite their vaguely similar banded patterns, this snake inhabits wetland areas usually avoided by copperheads. Note round pupils and absence of "pit."

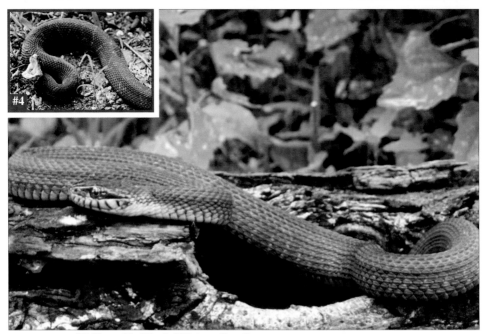

PHOTO #70 **Yellow Bellied Water Snake** *(Nerodia erythrogaster flavigaster)*
Inhabiting the same habitats as the Western Cottonmouth #4, *the Yellow Bellied Water Snake is similar in appearance to the darker versions of that snake. Note the round pupils and lack of "pit." Also note the uniform yellowish color of the belly, not seen on the cottonmouth.*

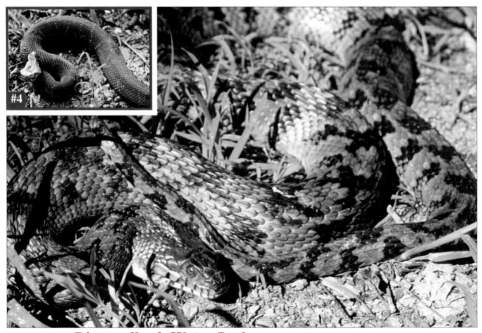

PHOTO #71 **Diamondback Water Snake** *(Nerodia rhombifer)*
This is a large, heavy-bodied water snake that inhabits the same regions and habitats as the Western Cottonmouth #4, *leading to its often being mistaken for that venomous species. Note the round pupils. Also note the lack of facial "pit" seen on the cottonmouth.*

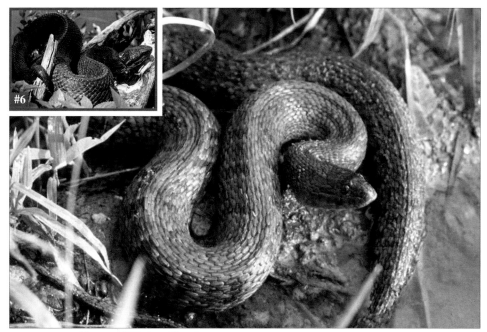

PHOTO #72 **Green Water Snake** *(Nerodia cyclopian)*
Another large, robust water snake that superficially resembles the Western Cottonmouth. The very similar Florida Green Water Snake (Nerodia floridana) *is often confused with the Florida Cottonmouth #6. Note the round pupils and lack of facial "pit."*

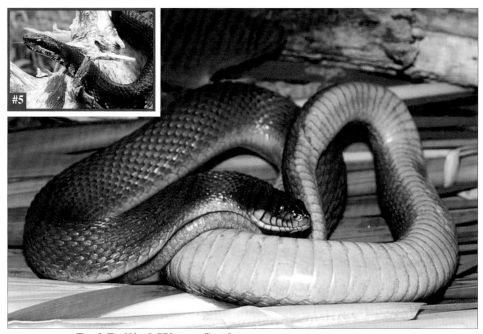

PHOTO #73 **Red Bellied Water Snake** *(Nerodia erythrogaster erythrogaster)*
Often confused with the Eastern Cottonmouth #5 with which it shares both range and habitat. Note the round pupils and absence of facial "pit." Also note the uniform reddish color on the belly, not seen on the cottonmouth.

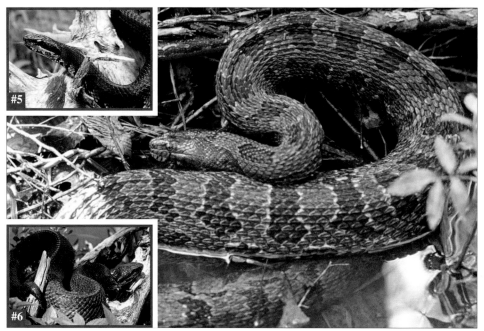

PHOTO #74 **Brown Water Snake** *(Nerodia taxispilota)*
This water snake's large size and stout body, along with its range and habitat preferences, lead to it often being confused with both the Eastern Cottonmouth #5 and the Florida Cottonmouth #6. *Note the round pupil and lack of facial "pit," which readily distinguish this harmless snake from the dangerous cottonmouths.*

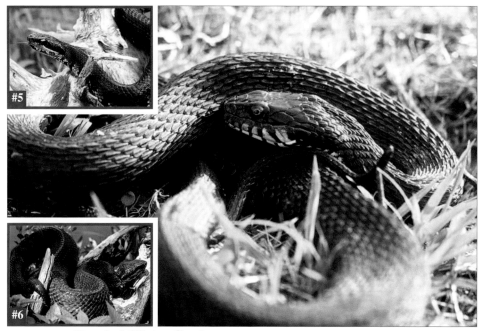

PHOTO #75 **Banded Water Snake** *(Nerodia fasciata fasciata)*
(dark phase) **Sometimes** confused with the Eastern #5 and Western Cottonmouths #6. *Note the round pupils and lack of facial "pit," both characteristics that distinguish this snake from the venomous cottonmouths.*

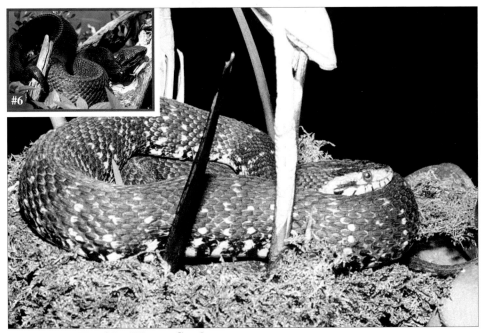

PHOTO #76 **Florida Water Snake** *(Nerodia fasciata picitiventris)*
(dark color phase) Often confused with the Florida Cottonmouth #6. Note the round as opposed to elliptical pupils and lack of facial "pit" seen on the cottonmouth.

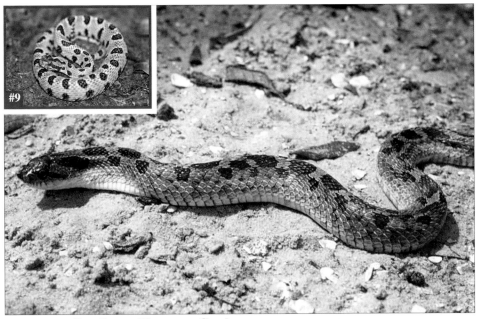

PHOTO #77 **Southern Hognose Snake** *(Heterodon simus)*
This snake's color scheme sometimes leads to it being confused with the Carolina Pygmy Rattlesnake #9. Note the presence of round as opposed to elliptical pupils, and the lack of a facial "pit," both characteristics that readily distinguish this species from the Pygmy Rattlesnake, as does the absense of a rattle on the tail.

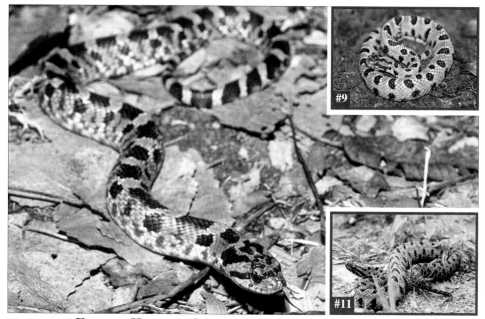

PHOTO #78 **Eastern Hognose Snake** *(Heterodon platyrhinos)*
The Eastern Hognose is a highly variable snake ranging in color from solid gray, olive, or black to a variety of spotted patterns highlighted by colors ranging from yellow to orange to red. Spotted individuals are sometimes confused with both the Carolina #9 and Western Pygmy Rattlesnakes #11, from which they may be told by their round pupils and lack of "pit," as well as by the more obvious absence of a rattle.

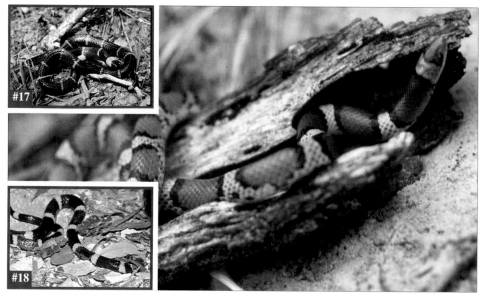

PHOTO #79 **Florida Scarlet Snake** *(Cemophora coccinea coccinea)*
The Florida Scarlet Snake, and the very similar Northern Scarlet Snake (C.c. coccinea), share their range with the Eastern Coral Snake #17 and are often confused with it. Both the Northern Scarlet Snake and the nearly identical Texas Scarlet Snake (C.c. lineri) can be found within the range of the Texas Coral Snake #18 and can be confused with that species as well. All Scarlet Snakes may be differentiated from all Coral Snakes by the fact that the nose of the Scarlet Snake is always red while the nose of the Coral Snake is always black.

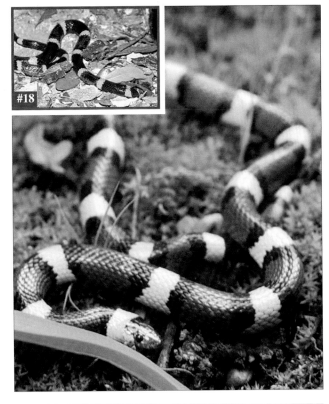

PHOTO #80
Scarlet Kingsnake
(Lampropeltis triangulum elapsoides)
This species is frequently mistaken for the Eastern Coral Snake, and its nearly identical cousins the Louisiana Milk Snake and the Mexican Milk Snake are often confused with the Texas Coral Snake #18. All can be told apart by the following rhyme, which refers to the arrangement of colors on the two snakes: "red touching yellow, kill a fellow" (refers to the Coral Snakes); "red touching black, venom lack" (refers to the harmless Scarlet Kingsnake and the Milk Snakes). These snakes can also be quickly told apart by the color of the snout, which is always red on the Scarlet Kingsnake and Milk Snakes and always black on the Coral Snakes.

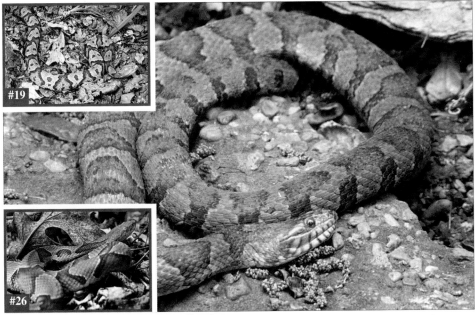

PHOTO #81 **Northern Water Snake** *(Nerodia sipedon sipedon)*
This snake's pattern of dark bands across the back causes it to sometimes be confused with the Osage and Southern Copperheads #19 & #26. Note that the bands on the Northern Water Snake are wide at the top and narrow on the sides, opposite of the copperhead whose bands are narrow at the top and wide at the sides. Also note round pupil and lack of "pit."

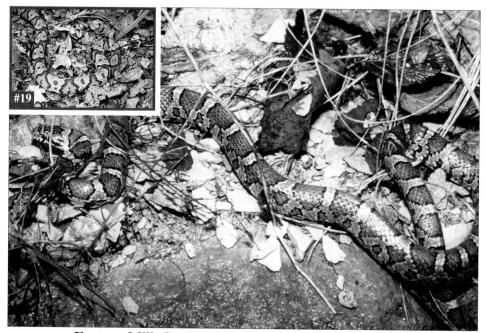

PHOTO #82 **Eastern Milk Snake** (*Lampropeltis triangulum triangulum*)
These harmless and useful snakes are often killed when mistaken for Northern Copperhead #19, from which they may be told by their round pupil and lack of facial "pit." Also note the dark markings on the back, which are in the form of blotches as opposed to bands seen on the copperhead.

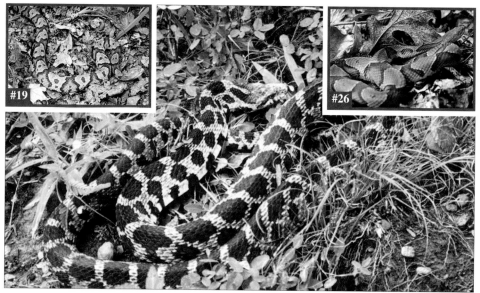

PHOTO #83 **Western Fox Snake** (*Elaphe vulpina vulpina*)
The russet color on the head of this snake causes many people to mistake it for a copperhead, in spite of the fact that most of the Fox Snake's range is well to the north of where any copperhead may be found. The range of the Fox Snake does overlap slightly with that of the Osage Copperhead #26 in parts of Missouri and Iowa, and with the Northern Copperhead #19 in a few places in Illinois. Note the round pupil and lack of facial "pit," both characteristics that distinguish this snake from the venomous copperhead.

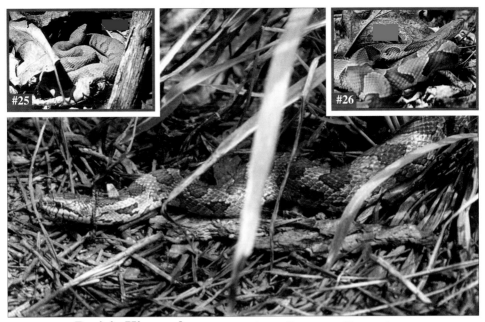

PHOTO #84 **Prairie Kingsnake** *(Lampropeltis calligaster calligaster)*
The author is at a loss to explain why this species is frequently mistaken for a copperhead. Perhaps it is because its dorsal blotches and head markings sometimes tend to be a russet color. As with most other harmless species in the United States, the Prairie Kingsnake possesses round pupils as opposed to elliptical pupils seen in pit vipers like the Northern Copperhead #25, and the Osage Copperhead #26, and lacks the facial "pit" which gives the venomous pit vipers their name.

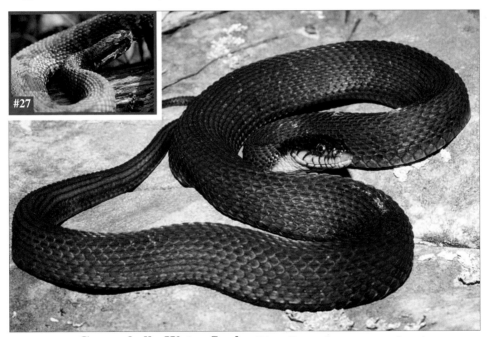

PHOTO #85 **Copperbelly Water Snake** *(Nerodia erythrogaster neglecta)*
The uniform dark dorsal coloration and aquatic habits both mimic the Western Cottonmouth #27, which shares a portion of its range with this species. Note the coppery color on the chin and face, never seen on a cottonmouth. Also note round pupils and lack of facial "pit."

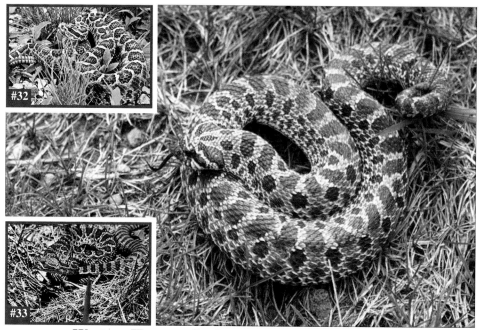

PHOTO #86 **Western Hognose Snake** *(Heterodon nasicus nasicus)*
The pattern of dorsal blotches on this snake is reminiscent of a number of rattlesnakes found within its range, including the **Western Massasauga #32, Desert Massasauga, and Prairie Rattlesnake #33.** *Note the lack of facial "pit" and the round pupil. Much more obvious is the lack of a rattle on the tail.*

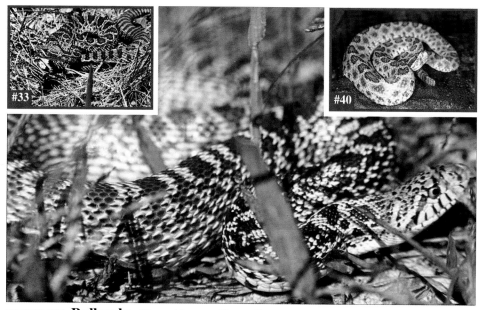

PHOTO #87 **Bullsnake** *(Pituophis catenifer sayi)*
Large and heavy bodied like many rattlesnakes, the Bullsnake is also possessed with a color and pattern that are similar in some respects. In addition, it has the habit of vibrating its tail when threatened, which in dry leaves or grass can produce a sound similar to a rattle. It is sometimes confused *with the* Prairie Rattlesnake #33 *and the* Western and Desert Massasaugas #40, *from which it may be most readily distinguished by the absence of a rattle on the tail. Also note round pupil and lack of "pit."*

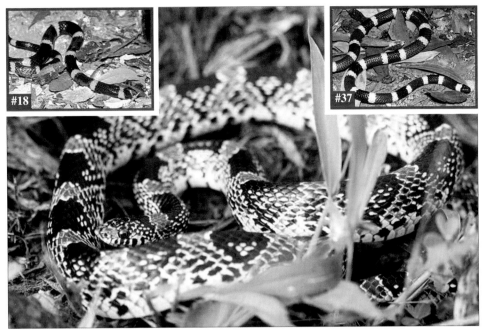

PHOTO #88 **Texas Long-Nosed Snake** *(Rhinocheilus lecontei lecontei)*
Because of a preponderance of red, black, and yellow pigmentation, this snake is occasionally confused with the Texas Coral Snake #18. An almost identical cousin, the Western Long-Nosed Snake may be confused with the Western Coral Snake #37. On the Long-nosed Snakes, however, the colors are diffused and do not form well-defined rings as on the Coral Snakes.

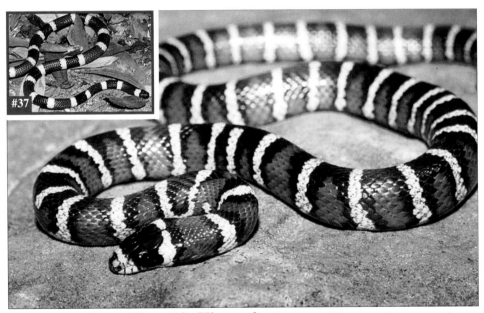

PHOTO #89 **Arizona Mountain Kingsnake** *(Lampropeltis pyromelana pyromelana)*
This handsome serpent may be easily confused with the Western Coral Snake #37, which shares much of its range. On the harmless Kingsnake, the snout is yellow or cream colored, while on the dangerous Coral the snout is black. The poem "red touches yellow, kill a fellow; red touches black, venom lack" applies to the arrangement of the red, yellow, and black rings and is a good way to differentiate between these two similar snakes.

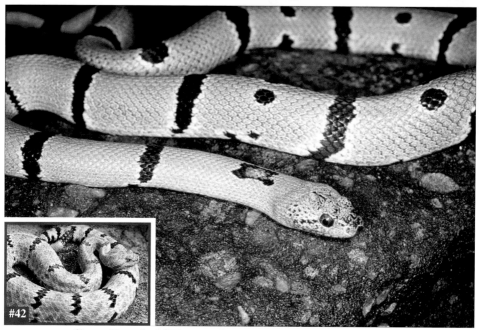

PHOTO #90 **Gray Banded Kingsnake** *(Lampropeltis alterna)*
This snake may at first glance be easily mistaken for the Mottled Rock Rattlesnake #42, which has a very similar color pattern, and occurs in many of the same areas. Note the round as opposed to elliptical pupil, the lack of a "pit," and the lack of a rattle on the tail.

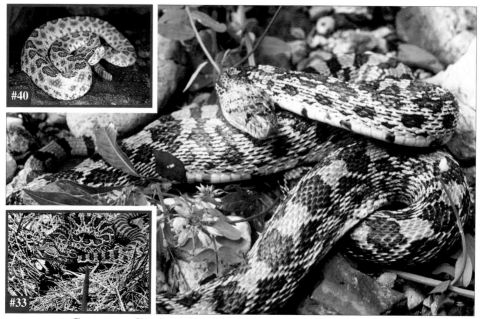

PHOTO #91 **Sonoran Gopher Snake** *(Pituophis catenifer affinis)*
This snake's color pattern of dorsal blotches coupled with a tail shaking behavior when threatened sometimes cause it to be confused with the Desert Massasauga #40 and the Prairie Rattlesnake #33 from which can be most readily distingushed by the absence of a rattle, as well as its round pupils and lack of "pit."

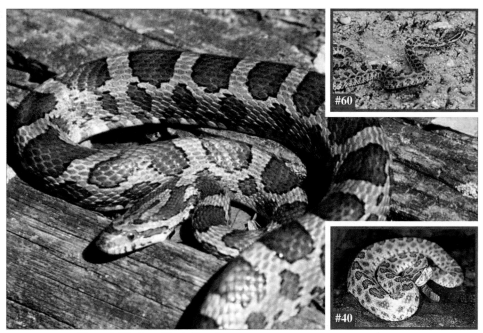

PHOTO #92 **Great Plains Rat Snake** *(Elaphe guttata emoryi)*
This snake's pattern of blotches on the back resembles the pattern on several types of rattlesnakes found within its range, including the Hopi Rattlesnake #60, Prairie Rattlesnake, and Desert Massasauga #40. Note the lack of a rattle, round pupils, and lack of "pit."

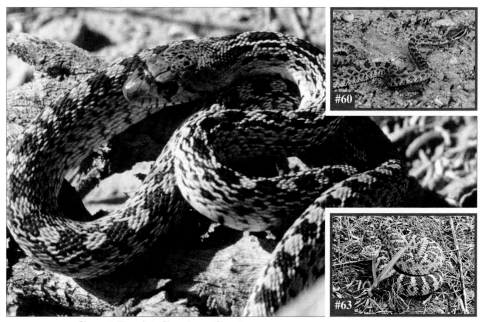

PHOTO #93 **Great Basin Gopher Snake** *(Pituophis catenifer deserticola)*
Dorsal blotches and tail shaking behavior may lead some to mistake this snake for a rattlesnake, four types of which occur within its range: the Hopi Rattlesnake #60, the Great Basin Rattlesnake, Midget Faded Rattlesnake, and the Northern Pacific Rattlesnake #63. Note the obvious lack of a rattle on the tail, round pupils, and lack of a facial "pit".

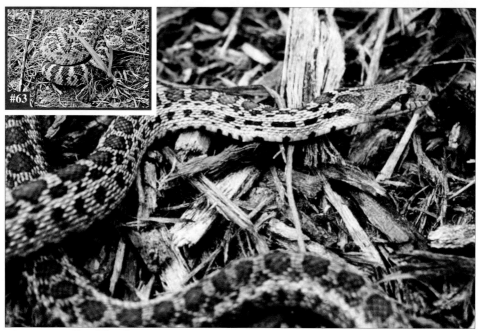

PHOTO #94 **Pacific Gopher Snake** *(Pituophis catenifer catenifer)*
Dorsal blotches and tail-shaking behavior occasionally lead to this snake being mistaken for the
Northern Pacific Rattlesnake #63 with which it shares both range and habitat. Note lack of rattle on the tail, round pupils, and lack of facial "pit."

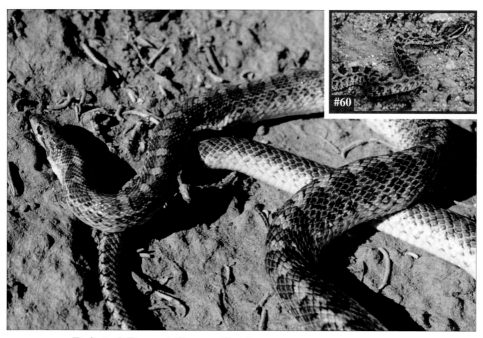

PHOTO #95 **Painted Desert Glossy Snake** *(Arizona elegans eburnata)*
Sometimes confused with the Hopi Rattlesnake #60 from which it may be distinguished by the lack of a rattle or a facial "pit," as well as the presence of a round as opposed to elliptical pupil.

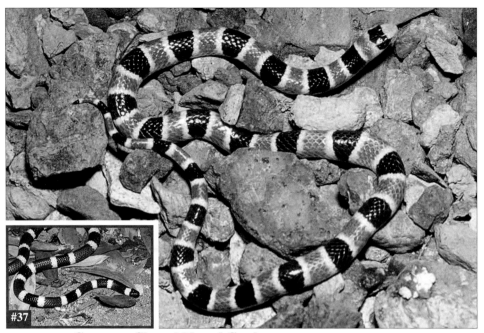

PHOTO #96 **Sonoran Shovel Nosed Snake** *(Chionactis palarostris)*
Most experts consider this snake to be a true *mimic of the Western Coral Snake #37, despite the fact that the colorful bands do not extend onto the belly, a characteristic by which this harmless species may be told from the dangerous Coral Snake.*

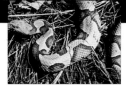

COPPERHEADS
(Agkistrodon contortrix)

There are five distinct subspecies of copperheads found in North America. Their range encompasses much of the highly populated eastern United States and in many regions they are our most common venomous snake, a combination of factors that lead to their being responsible for more venomous snakebites than any other snake in America.

Fortunately, the venom of copperheads is not highly toxic and deaths from their bite are extremely rare. Lest this statement be misunderstood, let me firmly state that the bite of a copperhead is a serious affair and requires immediate medical attention! Deaths from copperhead bites have been recorded, though most occurred many decades ago, before the advent of modern medical facilities. Venomous snakebite expert Dr. Sherman Minton reported in his 1969 book *Venomous Reptiles* that the fatality rate from copperhead bites was about .3 percent, and it is undoubtedly less than that today. Still, loss of fingers or toes or permanent crippling of a hand or foot are sometimes seen with copperhead bites; and a severe envenomation would likely prove to be one of the most painful and unpleasant experiences of one's life! With proper treatment, the survival rate today is probably 100 percent.

All copperheads are primarily woodland animals, though they may also be found in thickets and overgrown fields. They are particularly fond of derelict barns and buildings in overgrown areas, where they find both shelter and food. Like all pit vipers, copperheads give birth to fully formed young. The normal litter size is six to 12, usually born in late August or September. The 6- to 8-inch-long young are miniature replicas of the adults, except for a bright yellow tail tip which when wriggled resembles a small grub and is used to attract food within striking distance (see photo #20). Herpetologists have coined the phrase "caudal lure" to describe this special char-

RANGE OF THE COPPERHEAD IN THE UNITED STATES

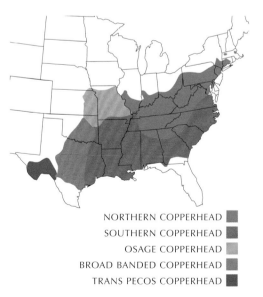

NORTHERN COPPERHEAD ■
SOUTHERN COPPERHEAD ■
OSAGE COPPERHEAD ■
BROAD BANDED COPPERHEAD ■
TRANS PECOS COPPERHEAD ■

acteristic that is shared by many other species of young pit vipers, including the cottonmouths.

Like many snake species, copperheads are primarily nocturnal animals, and especially during hotter summer months will spend the days hidden in hollow logs, stumps, or beneath rocks or leaf litter. Their cryptic color pattern of light brown with darker brown bands provides all five subspecies with exquisite camouflage and when lying among dead leaves on the forest floor, these snakes are almost invisible (see photo #19).

They prey on a wide variety of small vertebrates both warm- and cold-blooded and will also feed on many invertebrates. They are, in turn, preyed upon by a variety of predators, including birds of prey like the broad-winged hawk, a notorious snake killer that ranges in summer throughout much of the copperhead's range. A number of mammalian carnivores also prey on copperheads, the most significant of which is the opossum who possesses a high degree of resistance to snake venoms. But their greatest enemies other than man are other snakes, most especially the several varieties of kingsnakes with whom they share their range and who are also possessed with immunity to venom.

As is the case with many snakes, copperheads possess well-developed musk glands and when aroused they are capable of emitting a strong odor. Some people have likened this scent to the smell of cucumbers, and there is a widely held belief that the presence of copperheads in the woods may be ascertained by the detection of the smell of cucumbers. In truth, snakes only emit their musk when badly frightened; and the comparison of copperhead musk to the odor of cucumbers is subjective. To me, copperhead musk smells not like cucumbers but like, well, copperhead musk! Although I have personally experienced detecting musky odors similar to those produced by snakes while in the outdoors, I have never been able to positively link the odor to a nearby snake. I have on occasion been able to link the odor to a nearby plant. Many woodland plants produce flowers with a wide variety of smells, and most people who claim to be able to "smell copperheads" are I believe in fact detecting the odor of nearby plants.

See the map on the opposite page for an approximation of the ranges of the five races of copperheads. Additional information on the natural history of copperheads is provided on the following pages in the descriptions of the five individual subspecies.

Northern Copperhead

(subspecies *mokasen*)

PHOTO #19, 20 (RIGHT) & 25

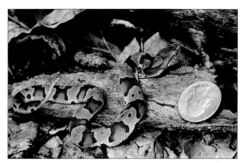

Like all other copperheads, the northern subspecies has a distinctive color pattern consisting of dark brown houglass-shaped bands on the back, sharply contrasting with the much lighter brown of the rest of the body, and a "coppery" colored head from which the snake derives its name. The exact shade of brown can be variable, but usually has a distinctively reddish hue. In this race of copperhead there are small dark spots present on the side of the body between the hourglass bands, which is one of the characters that defines this northern subspecies. A lover of upland woods, the northern copperhead is most common throughout the Appalachian Mountains and Cumberland Plateau and in much of this area it is a very common snake. In the rest of its range it is locally common on wooded ridges and upland woods. It may also be found in valleys and wooded creek bottoms, but avoids swamps and wetlands.

Northern copperheads are one of the largest of the five subspecies, with mature adults averaging from $2^1/2$ feet (females) to $3^1/2$ feet or larger (males). The record length according to published literature is 53 inches; however, I have personally seen a specimen, which for many years was exhibited at the nature station in Land Between the Lakes National Recreation Area (western Kentucky), that measured an incredible 58 inches. I have seen a number of specimens from that area that were in excess of 40 inches. Like many other pit vipers, male northern copperheads are larger than females and all the really large individuals I have seen were males. Large males sometimes engage in a fascinating behavior known as "male combat." Two male snakes of equal size will crawl parallel to one another with the anterior third of the body raised several inches off the ground, entwining the raised portion of their bodies as they attempt to force their opponent's head to the ground. They never employ the use of their fangs and the entire contest is essentially a wrestling match from which both winner and loser emerge unscathed. Male rattlesnakes and cottonmouths also routinely engage in this behavior, which is undoubtedly territorial in nature.

Abandoned barns and derelict buildings that have collapsed are a favorite haunt for these and other snakes that find both food and shelter there. Mice and small rodents are a primary food for adults, though lizards and frogs may also be eaten along with the young of ground-nesting birds. Insects and other invertebrates are probably a staple for newborns (I have fed captive born copperheads earthworms). Adults will also eat some insects, especially cicadas, which they seem to relish. The ringneck snake (a small, harmless species common throughout the northern copperhead's range) is reportedly a favorite food item for juveniles.

Their enemies include most predatory animals that share their range, including, of course, other snakes like the kingsnakes that specialize in eating their own kind and possess an immunity to snake venoms. I once watched as another snake, a black racer, killed and ate a small northern copperhead. Since black racers are not immune to snake venom, the attacking racer was at some risk. Grasping the much smaller victim by the head with lightning speed, the racer immediately began to violently thrash its body against the ground while methodically chewing on the head. After about two minutes the hapless young copperhead was quite dead and was swallowed by his much larger cousin.

I have seen a number of snakebites by this subspecies, and most cases recovered fully without any permanent damage. However, copperhead venom contains powerful digestive enzymes that can destroy a lot of tissue at the site of the bite. Jim Harrison, herpetologist and toxicologist from the Kentucky Reptile Zoo, suffered what is perhaps the worst northern copperhead bite with which I am personally familiar. A large, 3½-foot snake angrily embedded both fangs into his left middle finger. The amount of tissue damage was so great that the finger eventually had to be amputated.

I have had more personal experience with this snake than perhaps any other venomous species, having collected or observed in the wild and captivity many hundreds of specimens over the years. In the 600-square-mile Land Between the Lakes National Recreation Area of western Kentucky and west Tennessee, the northern copperhead is one of the most common snake species. The area consists mostly of deciduous upland forest, and is prime habitat for these snakes. They are similarly widespread and common throughout the Cumberland Plateau and the Appalachian Mountains.

When hunting these snakes in the spring, I look for fallen-down barns or outbuildings, or old homesteads with pieces of roofing tin or boards strewn about. Such places will nearly always yield copperheads, as well as other snakes. In midsummer, "road hunting" at night, especially after a rain, is most productive. In August, gravid females move into brush piles or stacks of undisturbed boards or lumber, old collapsed wooden buildings, etc., to await birthing. In the area of my home in far western Kentucky this habit of seeking out a secure location for birthing leads to many human encounters with this snake.

Local farmers here grow a variety of tobacco that requires a period of curing during which the tobacco plants are hung in a barn and cured with heat from smoldering fires in the barn floor. This process, known as "firing," requires the use of large amounts of what is known as "slab lumber", which is actually the first few cuts made from a fresh log at the sawmill. These "slabs" are delivered in large truckloads and dumped near the tobacco barns that are located in rural areas, often in or near the woodlands that are home to the copperhead.

Pregnant female copperheads seeking a safe refuge will burrow deep into the labyrinth of crevices created by the loosely stacked lumber. The timing of the tobacco "firing" process in late summer and early fall coincides with the birthing time of baby copperheads. When beginning the "firing" of his crop, many a tobacco farmer has encountered a litter of baby copper-heads often still accompanied by their mother. In spite of these encounters between man and snake, bites to tobacco farmers are actually rare, a testimony to the normally docile nature of the copperhead. At this same time in late summer and early fall, activity for all snake species begins to increase as these cold-blooded animals seek suitable hibernating places in which to spend the winter. At this time of year, "road cruising" can be a productive method of observing these normally shy and reclu-sive snakes.

Southern Copperhead
(subspecies *contortrix*)
PHOTO #2 & 3 (right)

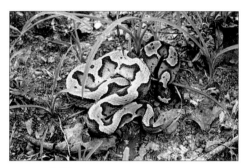

Similar in size (record length 52 inch-es) and in most other respects to the northern copperhead, but the small dark spots between the crossbands tend to be diminished or lacking altogether, and there is a sharper contrast between the light and dark pigments. Individuals from the Deep South are among the most beau-tiful of the copperheads, often with hues of bright orange or yellow, which sharply contrast with the darker crossbars.

For detailed information on the natu-ral history of the southern copperhead, the reader is referred to the species account on preceding pages. Also read the account for the northern copperhead, as the two subspecies are almost identi-cal in most aspects of their natural histo-ry. Like the northern race, the southern copperhead is locally common and in prime habitats can reach the same kind of population densities seen with its northern cousin. I have collected and observed many specimens of southern copperhead over the years in the Ozarks of northern Arkansas and southern Missouri, as well as in west Tennessee, North and South Carolina, and Georgia.

The most strikingly beautiful speci-mens of this race are reputed to come from the rare population that exists in two counties in the Florida panhandle. While employed at the Ross Allen Reptile Institute in Silver Springs, Florida, in the early 1970s, I was fortu-nate enough to see a couple of these specimens and they are indeed hand-some snakes. But I have also seen speci-mens from the "Sandhills" region of South Carolina that rival the beauty of the Florida specimens.

Recent studies of snake venoms indi-cate that the venom of the southern cop-perhead may be more toxic than that of the northern subspecies. I was once bit-ten by a 2-foot female on the tip of my right ring finger. Although only one fang was imbedded, it was a "feeding strike" and a large amount of venom was inject-ed. While I never experienced any symp-toms of systemic poisoning, the local symptoms were pronounced. The swelling eventually encompassed the entire arm, and the tissues at the site of the bite became necrotic and sloughed, leaving a paralyzed and deadened finger-tip consisting mostly of scar tissue. Although I never considered the bite to be life threatening, I was impressed and alarmed by the severity of the pain at the site of the bite. While I have experienced much more serious bites by other species, I don't recall any that were as painful. Other individuals I have known who have experienced numerous snakebites confirm my observations about the discomfort associated with copperhead bites.

Osage Copperhead
(subspecies *phaeogaster*)
PHOTO #1 & 26 (right)

This subspecies is found in the northern Ozark Plateau across most of Missouri and into the Flint Hills region of eastern Kansas, being quite common in many areas. Osage copperheads closely resemble the southern subspecies in appearance, the most obvious difference being the presence of a thin white line border-ing the dark crossbands and an over-all browner coloration. This race is not appreciably different from the northern and southern subspecies in natural history, and the reader is referred to the species account on pages 84-85 for general information about the natural history of this sub-species. Also read the account for the northern copperhead, as the two sub-species are not appreciably different in their biology. Osage copperheads are somewhat smaller, the recorded maximum length being 40 inches. Much of this snake's range in the Ozarks of Missouri is very similar to that of its northern cousin, being mostly upland woods, but this race also ranges westward into the tall grass prairie region of eastern

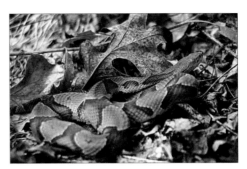

Kansas, where the deciduous wood-lands of the eastern United States begin to give way the open expanse of the plains. Even here, the Osage copperhead is primarily a forest species, never found far from wood-land areas.

I recently took a trip to the Missouri Ozarks with my youngest son expressly to find and photograph an Osage copper-head. After a nearly five-hour drive from our home in western Kentucky, we were well within the range of our quarry. At the very first stop we made near a small stream, my son discovered a small female coiled among the leaf litter not 50 feet from the truck. In less than five min-utes of snake hunting, we had accom-plished our goal! Such remarkable suc-cess in locating a serpent in its natural habitat is rarely so easy, but gives a good indication of how common these snakes can be in ideal habitats. In several other excursions to the wilds of both the Missouri Ozarks and eastern Kansas, I have seen only two additional specimens, thus, the author's personal experience with this subspecies in the wild is quite limited. For additional reading on this subspecies, I recommend *The Amphibians and Reptiles of Missouri* by Tom Johnson, and *Amphibians and Reptiles in Kansas* by Joseph Collins.

Broad Banded Copperhead
(subspecies laticinctus)
PHOTO #31

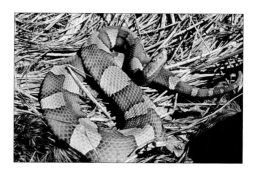

As its name implies, this race is distinguished from other copperheads by the characteristically broader dark bands across the back. Broad banded copperheads are found from north-central Oklahoma southward in a wide band through central Texas. Their preferred habitat is the oak woodlands that are interspersed through the southern prairies. In the drier areas of their range they are restricted to river valleys and bottomlands that support the growth of trees. The natural history is similar to that of the other subspecies. In size they average somewhat smaller than the Northern, Southern, and Osage races, being no more than 3 feet in length. The record length is 37^1/$_2$ inches.

These copperheads are locally very common in prime habitats in the woodlands of central Texas. Once while visiting a roadside reptile display in north-central Texas, I witnessed a snake hunter bring in his catch from the last few nights of "road cruising."

He had about a dozen broad banded copperheads along with a few western diamondback rattlesnakes that he sold to the proprietor. This encounter, along with a half-dozen or so captive specimens held over the years, constitutes the sum of the author's first-hand experience with this race. For more information on this subspecies, the reader may wish to pick up a copy of *Poisonous Snakes of Texas* by Andrew Price.

Trans-Pecos Copperhead

(subspecies *pictigaster*)

PHOTO #57

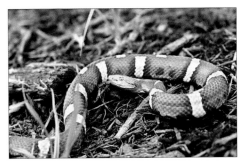

As its name implies, this race lives in the Trans-Pecos area of Texas, including the Big Bend region, and it is the most westerly occurring subspecies of the copperhead. Unlike its relatives to the north and east, the Trans-Pecos copperhead ranges into true desert. But even here, its preferred habitats are the mountain canyons and draws that support the growth of oak and pine. Within this snake's range in the arid and inhospitable Chihuahuan Desert, there are canyons and mountains containing oasis of woodlands, sometimes with small streams that trickle rather than flow but provide a "microhabitat" similar to that found in much of the eastern United States. In fact, the Trans-Pecos copperhead is considered to be a "relict" animal, left over from a time about 11.000 years ago when the Chihuahuan Desert was deciduous woodland. The Chisos Mountains in Big Bend National Park con-tain some prime examples of "relict" habitats suitable for this snake.

This is the smallest of the five races of copperheads, averaging only about 2 feet in length. The record length is 33 inches. In color and pattern, they are very handsome snakes, exhibiting a rich chestnut hue that is overall much darker than that of other subspecies. The dark, hourglass bands are as wide as those of the broad banded copperhead, but are dramatically highlighted by a white or light yellow crescent in the center of the band. As might be expected from an animal that has adapted to a habitat that has changed radically from its origins, this subspecies of copperhead has less in common with its more easterly relatives. The primary food is lizards, which are extremely common in the desert environment, but they will also readily eat mice and other prey.

The reproductive rate for these snakes is apparently lower than its eastern cousins. Three captive born litters from two females in my possession at the Woods & Wetlands Wildlife Center numbered three, four, and four. Interestingly, the young were larger and more robust than newborn southern or northern copperheads. They were also at birth much darker in color than their parents, slowly getting lighter and richer in color as they grew.

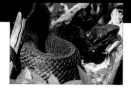

COTTONMOUTHS
(Agkistrodon piscivorous)

Also widely known as "water moccasin," the cottonmouths are to many the most feared and dreaded residents of the cypress and Tupelo swamps of the Deep South.

Though they are quite dangerous and capable of inflicting a fatal bite, their venom is not as potent as that of most rattlesnakes and their reputation as aggressive animals prone to attack is grossly exaggerated. However, unlike most snakes that flee from an approaching human, the cottonmouth does tend to stand its ground, and if sufficiently provoked, may strike savagely and repeatedly. Though fatalities from cottonmouths are an uncommon occurrence, numerous deaths from cottonmouth bites have been recorded, including some in recent years. Their venom is more toxic than that of their cousins the copperheads, and often produces large amounts of tissue damage due to the powerful digestive enzymes present in the venom. Specimens of this snake from the Deep South can attain an impressive size (up to 6 feet), and such animals can deliver a large dose of venom. In summation, this is not a snake to be messing with!

There are three very similar subspecies of cottonmouths found in North America. The differences between the races are so subtle as to be apparent only to an expert. All three are similar in habits and habitat, being decidedly aquatic animals. Their favorite haunts are swamps and marshes, including brackish waters and occasionally salt marshes. They may also be found along the banks of creeks and rivers, as well as lakes and ponds, the latter more so in the southern parts of their range. Though closely tied to water, they may sometimes wander great distances from its source.

Cottonmouths feed on a wide variety of animals, including fish, frogs, salamanders, small mammals, birds, and even young turtles and baby alligators. They

RANGE OF THE COTTONMOUTHS IN THE UNITED STATES

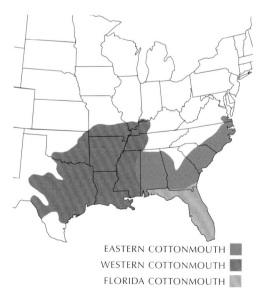

EASTERN COTTONMOUTH
WESTERN COTTONMOUTH
FLORIDA COTTONMOUTH

also readily eat other snakes, which explains why they are almost never seen in the company of the harmless water snakes that are abundant in the same habitats and locales. They are not above scavenging and will eat dead flesh that is bordering on putrid.

The enemies of cottonmouths are not as numerous as with many snakes. Kingsnakes will use their immunity to venom to prey on young and juvenile cottonmouths but the large adults are safe from most kingsnakes. Predatory fishes such as bass are also known to feed on young cottonmouths on rare occasions. Raptorial birds no doubt kill a few, and some wading birds like the great blue heron have been known to eat the smaller individuals. The heron uses it stiletto-like beak to repeatedly stab snakes to death and has also been seen picking up snakes and violently slamming them against a log or tree trunk. In the Deep South, adult alligators no doubt pose a significant threat, and throughout their range the Virginia Opossum, the most notorious snake-eating mammal in America, is probably one of this snake's worst enemies. Raccoons may also be predators, especially of the young. I know of one instance where a raccoon in the wild fed on the body of a recently killed cottonmouth, though interestingly, it did not eat the head.

Cottonmouths are closely related to the copperheads and in many respects they may be considered a lowland, aquatic version of the copperhead. They share many of the same characteristics of their biology and behavior. Adult male cottonmouths engage in "male combat" behavior (see description of

northern copperhead), and like the copperheads, cottonmouths are livebearers, giving birth to an average of six to 10 fully formed young in late August through September. Newborn cottonmouths may be 8 to 10 inches long at birth and bear a close resemblance to their cousins the copperheads, being strongly marked with a distinct pattern of hourglass-shaped dark bands across the back (see photo #7). They also possess the bright yellow tail tip that is used as a lure (see account of the copperheads). The banded pattern of the young fades with age, and adults gradually take on darker colors as they mature.

Adults in the wild often become stained from immersion in muddy, silt-laden waters. I have seen individuals that were a uniform muddy brown, reddish brown, or dark gray, depending on the soil type where they lived. If taken into captivity, these same snakes will regain their original color after one or two sheddings of the skin. The appearance of a freshly shed adult can vary from almost solid black to olive green. On some specimens a distinct remnant of the youthful bands will remain evident. For a more complete description of the color and pattern of this snake, see the accounts for the three subspecies given on the following pages.

The name "cottonmouth" is derived from this species' peculiar habit of opening the mouth when frightened or threatened, revealing the white membrane lining the inside of the mouth (see photo #4). Though a few non-venomous snakes also sometimes exhibit this "gaping" behavior as part of a "threat display," no other aquatic snake species is known to do so. Thus any snake seen in wetland habitat within the cottonmouth's range, that "gapes" may be reasonably assumed to be a cottonmouth. The cottonmouths share their range with many other aquatic snake species; in fact, there are several dozen types of snakes native to the United States that live in and around water. But the cottonmouths are America's only venomous aquatic snakes. Several species of harmless water snakes in America (genus Nerodia) closely resemble the cottonmouths in color, pattern, and body form, and these snakes present for most people the most difficult identification challenge of all our pit vipers.

For photographs of some harmless water snakes that are often confused with the cottonmouth, see the section of this book titled "Photos of Non-Venomous Mimics." Photos 70, 71, 72, 73, 74, 75 and 76 are all harmless water snakes that may be confused with the cottonmouth.

Cottonmouths in the wild may be distingusihed from the harmless water snakes by the way in which both swim. Cottonmouths are much more buoyant in the water, floating as if made of cork, while the harmless water snakes ride much lower in the water, with just the top of the back above the surface. When swimming, the cottonmouths also hold the head up higher, an inch or two above the surface, while the harmless water snakes swim with the head resting on the surface. These are admittedly subtle differences that, while they may be readily apparent to an expert, are not so easily discerned by the layman. Also important to note is the fact that cottonmouths and harmless water snakes can and do swim occasionally below the surface, and both may appear with just the head sticking out of the water.

Incidentally, cottonmouths can bite underwater, despite the widely held myth to the contrary. Of the many myths and fantastic tales told about snakes, one of my favorites is the story of the water skier (or boater, or fisherman, etc) who fell into a "nest" or "ball" of cottonmouths and died almost immediately after being savagely bitten hundreds of times. The only thing in this story that is remotely true is the fact that hundreds of bites by cottonmouths would undoubtedly prove fatal! First, cottonmouths do not congregate into a concentrated mass such as described in this fantasy, and if they did it would not be in the middle of a large body of open water, as these are animals of creeks, swamps, and marshes. When they do occur in lakes and ponds, they restrict their activities to the shallow waters of the shores and banks. This tale is so widespread that it may be heard in regions where cottonmouths are not even found. I have been told this story on a number of occasions, once by a rancher from South Dakota, never mind that the nearest cottonmouth to be found in the wild would have been several hundred miles away!

Western Cottonmouth

(subspecies *leucostoma*)

PHOTO #4 (right) & 27

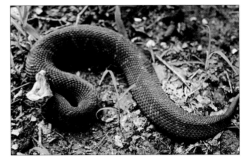

T his is the smallest subspecies of cottonmouths, rarely exceeding 4 feet in length, though the record is 5 feet, 2 inches. Like most pit vipers, the males attain the largest size and any over 3 feet in length are invariably males. Generally speaking, western cottonmouths tend to be darker over-all than their eastern and Florida cousins; this is especially true of the facial markings, which on the western race are brown as opposed to white or cream. The overall color of freshly molted adults ranges from a dark olive green with black crossbands to an almost solid black above. As previously mentioned in the species account, many specimens from murky waters will be stained brown, reddish, or grayish, depending on the type of silt present in the water.

Of the three subspecies of cotton-mouths, I am most familiar with this race, having collected or observed in the wild many hundreds of specimens over the years. Most of my experiences with this snake have come in cypress swamps of the Mississippi Delta region of far western Kentucky and west Tennessee. Generally speaking, western cotton-mouths in the more northerly parts of their range tend to occur only locally and in disjunct populations. This is especially true in west Kentucky, southern Illinois and southeast Missouri. Where they do occur here, however, they can be quite common. If the habitat is protected by law or by remote and difficult access, these snakes, unmolested by humans can reach a population density probably not surpassed

by any other American pit viper, except perhaps the large congrega-tions of certain rattlesnake species that can occur at hibernating areas.

These snakes are prone to a gregari-ous nature. I once counted two dozen western cottonmouths sunning on a 30-foot section of log in a small cypress swamp in western Kentucky. Oddly, while continuing to explore the surround-ing swamp, I located only two more indi-viduals. On another occasion in this same area, I peered into a small hollow in a floating cypress log and found it tightly packed with four adults.

During the heyday of the U.S. Army Corps of Engineers, which covered sever-al decades beginning after World War II, countless acres of wetlands in the Mississippi valley were dredged and drained, significantly impacting on wet-land animals and plants of all variety. In recent years, the trend has been towards preservation of wetlands and in the region of my home in western Kentucky, these snakes are probably more numerous today than a few decades ago.

Throughout the Deep South, these snakes are widespread and common, being found in creeks, rivers, lakes, and ponds as well as in swamps and marsh-land. In southern Mississippi I have found them in clear, sandy-bottomed creeks, and in southern Alabama I once found a small pond no larger than a swimming pool and surrounded by agricultural land that was home to at least a half-dozen of these snakes. In the southern Ozark Mountains of northern Arkansas, I have seen them in cold mountain streams. All these scenarios are in stark contrast to where these snakes can be found near my stomping grounds in western Kentucky, where they are restricted mostly to swamps and marshes.

In late summer (mid-August), gravid females show a preference for beaver lodges as a place for birthing the young. The tangle of piled-up sticks of the lodge provide the baby snakes with a readily accessible escape from enemies and some will overwinter there. Females that give birth later (in late September or early October) may already be at the winter hibernating den, which may be some distance from water. Many western cottonmouths leave the swamps and lowlands each fall and overwinter in higher ground, which at times may be as much as a half-mile from water. Babies born here emerge the next spring and have to make the long trek back to the swamp.

When I was 17 years old I experienced my first venomous snakebite, inflicted by a three-day-old baby western cottonmouth that embedded one fang in the tip of my left index finger. The pronounced burning pain was immediately followed by swelling and discoloration at the site of the injection. The swelling progressed over the next few hours to the forearm and the tip of the finger turned from purple to black. It took several weeks for the tip of the finger to completely heal after a good chunk of skin and underlying tissue sloughed, leaving a permanent scar that remained in evidence until quite recently, when the results of the bite of a 4-foot alligator forever obscured the mark left by the little cottonmouth. Though the bite by the baby cottonmouth was inconsequential and as venomous snakebites go, was quite minor, it did leave me thinking about what damage a fully-grown adult could do!

My old snake hunting buddy, Mr. Kenny Maddox of Jackson, Tennessee, suffered what was perhaps the worst-case scenario of a cottonmouth bite. On a snake hunting trip to Reelfoot Lake in northwest Tennessee in the late 1960s he slipped and fell on a 2-foot western cottonmouth, whereupon the snake promptly bit him on the hip. Hurriedly grasping the snake, he desperately flung it into the air only to have it come down on his back and proceed to bite him again on the shoulder. This time the snake was thrown to the ground directly in front of him, but in his haste to escape he slipped in the mud and fell on it for a second time. The cottonmouth once again registered its distain for such intimacy with a human by biting him a third time, this time in the thigh. After finally escaping the jaws of the snake, Kenny was rushed by two companions to a hospital about 45 minutes away, where large doses of antivenin and trauma therapy pulled him through.

After some two weeks in the hospital he emerged with a harrowing and somewhat comical tale of how not to catch cottonmouths, and earned himself the distinction of being a foremost authority on "mud wrestling cottonmouths." Kenny sometimes still boasts that he cannot be killed by a cottonmouth, having survived the worst of what a cottonmouth can do to a human. But in his heart he knows that he is alive today by the grace of God and a heroic effort by his doctors and modern medicine, and I have noticed since that time a slightly more measured and cautious approach in his dealings with these snakes. Incidentally, the cottonmouth got away.

Eastern Cottonmouth

(subspecies piscivorous)

PHOTO #5

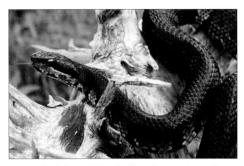

In habits and habitat this race is similar to the western cottonmouth. It differs chiefly in size, having a record length of 6 feet 2 inches, and large males can easily reach 5 feet. In color and pattern, this subspecies is much lighter than the western race, often being an olive green with dark crossbands, or light brown with darker brown to black bands. Eastern cottonmouths have a tendency to retain the banded pattern of the juvenile, and most specimens will show evidence of a banded pattern.

This race is common in wetland habitats throughout its range (see map). I have seen them in the wild only in the coastal plain of North Carolina, where I found them in typical cottonmouth habitats. For additional information regarding the natural history of this race, see the account given for cottonmouths in general and also review the account of both the Western Cottonmouth and the Florida Cottonmouth. An additional source of authoritative data on this race is available in the book *Reptiles of North Carolina* by Palmer and Braswell.

Florida Cottonmouth

(subspecies conanti)

PHOTO #6 & 7 (right)

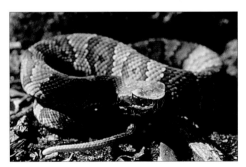

For information on the natural history of this subspecies, see the account for cottonmouths in general, and also refer to the account for the Western Cottonmouth. The most readily distinguishable difference between this race and its two cousins are the lighter facial markings and the presence of two dark vertical stripes on the snout. Photo #6 provides a good illustration of these "rostral stripes" which readily distinguish this subspecies. Large old individuals of this race are sometimes quite dark, being almost solid black dorsally. These snakes attain a huge size, equaling that of the eastern cottonmouth and averaging perhaps a bit larger. The record length is 6 feet 2½ inches. In the early 1970s, while employed at the Ross Allen Reptile Institute in Silver Springs, Florida, the author once caught a dozen Florida cottonmouths in one afternoon, all of which totaled 48 in length collectively! That's an average of 4 feet each. During my tenure at the institute, and later at the Saint Augustine Alligator Farm in St. Augustine, I personally observed several specimens that were in excess of 5 feet and at least a half-dozen that were within a few inches of the record. Sadly, for those few of us who value such creatures, behemoths like these are now quite uncommon.

The name "Florida" cottonmouth is appropriate for this subspecies, as it occurs mostly within that state (see range map). It is widespread, being found in probably every county, although it is apparently absent from the Florida Keys and according to one expert may be locally nonexistent. "Their populations tend to vary, with large areas of apparently prime habitat being entirely devoid of these reptiles," writes expert Alan Tennant in his book *A Field Guide to the Snakes of Florida.*

In many areas it is still a common serpent, though not as common as a few decades ago. Its habitat, like all cottonmouths, is aquatic and semiaquatic environments including river swamps, stream banks, marshes, wet prairies, lakes, and ponds. It may also be found in brackish water and salt marshes, including barrier islands. This race seems less tied to water than the other two subspecies and some-

times is found in dry environments, though it should be noted that within its range, water is a common and widespread element, and it is rare to find a place that is not near some water anywhere in the state.

The author has hunted these snakes mostly in central Florida along the Silver River and the Oklawaha River, where they show a preference for patches of saw grass bordering the riverbanks. In such places, they are often quite gregarious and several individuals can often be found in a single patch of saw grass in close proximity to one another. By contrast, in wet prairies and swamps, they seem more scattered and widespread. In the highlands of the Ocala National Forest I have found them in small ponds surrounded by large tracts of the dry "scrub" that characterizes much of that area. Oddly, I have captured a number of individuals that were severely emaciated, some of which died shortly after the stress of capture. Some experts have reported that parasite infestation is often heavy in this subspecies, which may provide an explanation.

The large size of this subspecies makes it a dangerous snake. The largest individuals may possess a quantity of venom up to three or four times the amount needed to kill a human. The venom is highly hemorrhagic and contains powerful digestive enzymes. As if this weren't enough, cottonmouth bites often result in infection with pathogenic bacteria present in both the mouth and venom. In the early 1970s, I met an individual who had been bitten years before on the lower leg. Most of the muscle tissue of the calf had been lost, resulting in permanent crippling.

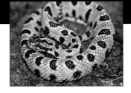

PYGMY RATTLESNAKES
(Sistrurus miliarius)

Our smallest rattlesnake species, *Sistrurus miliarius,* is represented in America by three subspecies. Most are less than 18 inches long, though one race may rarely reach a length of nearly 3 feet. Their rattle is so tiny that it is apparent only upon close examination, and it cannot be heard for a distance of more than a few feet.

Pygmy rattlesnakes, along with their larger but similar cousins the massasauga rattlesnakes *(Sistrurus catenatus)* are in many ways intermediate between America's other two pit viper genera *Agkistrodon* (copperheads and cottonmouths) and *Crotalus* (true rattlesnakes). Unlike the larger rattlesnakes, *Sistrurus* rattlers have large, plate-like scales on the top of the head, like those seen on the copperheads and cottonmouths, while on the larger "true rattlesnakes," the top of the head is covered with small scales.

Baby pygmy rattlers also have a bright yellow tail tip, the "caudal lure," which is discussed in the account of the copperheads, another indication of their kinship to the *Agkistrodon*. Newborns are so tiny that their coil is about the same diameter as a dime, and their brood size will usually average about six to eight; though much larger litters have been reported.

The venom of these diminutive rattlesnakes is fairly toxic, but their small size and subsequent small amounts of venom they inject make them much less dangerous than the larger rattlesnakes. They are not considered capable of inflicting a fatal bite and despite numerous cases of snakebite by this species, no human deaths have been recorded. Nonetheless, the bite of a pygmy rattler can be a serious affair and if untreated can lead to complications such as infection and gangrene. Some victims of pygmy rattler bites suffer permanent damage from tissue destruction, especially on extremities like fingers or toes.

Pygmy rattlesnakes are found in a variety of habitats throughout the south-

RANGE OF THE PYGMY RATTLE-SNAKE IN THE UNITED STATES

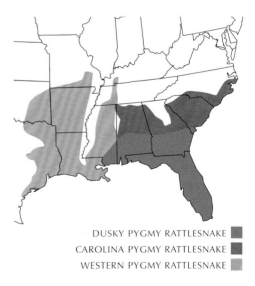

DUSKY PYGMY RATTLESNAKE ■
CAROLINA PYGMY RATTLESNAKE ■
WESTERN PYGMY RATTLESNAKE ■

eastern United States, but with the exception of some areas in Florida, they are usually not very common. As a general rule, these small rattlesnakes are fond of moist habitats such as damp woodlands or the edges of swamps and marshes. Baby pygmy rattlers are quite tiny, being only about 6 inches in length. Their color

and pattern mimic that of the adults, but are perhaps a bit brighter and more distinct.

Adults feed on mice, lizards, frogs, and salamanders as well as a variety of invertebrates, the latter being undoubtedly a staple for the young that are too small to swallow most vertebrate prey.

Carolina Pygmy Rattlesnake
(subspecies *miliarius*)
PHOTO #8 (right) & 9

Of the three races of pygmy rattlers, this subspecies is the most variable in color. Most specimens are light gray with dark brown or black blotches on the back. In between each dark blotch is a smaller reddish brown spot. The sides are also marked with dark spots. (See photo #8.) In a small area of coastal North Carolina around Pamlico Sound, a bright reddish color phase of this snake occurs. (See photo #9.)

The record length for this subspecies according to the *Peterson Field Guide to Reptiles and Amphibians of Eastern and Central North America* by Roger Conant and Joseph Collins is given as 25 inches, but William Palmer and Alvin Braswell in their book *Reptiles of North Carolina* report a specimen of just a fraction under 30 inches. Most individuals will be around 18 to 20 inches as adults. Like all three subspecies, this race of pygmy rattler is a feisty little snake when threatened. They will strike repeatedly and with lightning speed, though their strike is quite short,

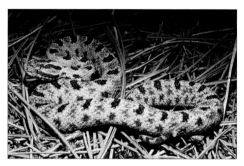

having a reach of only a few inches.

These little rattlers are apparently uncommon throughout most of their range, and I have never personally seen one in the wild. I did spend one night "road cruising" for the now rare red phase on the southern Albemarle peninsula in North Carolina, but was not fortunate enough to see one. Herpetologist Dale McGinnity, curator of ectotherms at the Nashville Zoo, maintains a collection of this rare color phase for captive breeding, and he generously supplied the photo of the red phase Carolina pygmy that appears in this book (photo #9). For additional information on the biology of the Carolina pygmy rattlesnake, read the preceding account given for pygmy rattlesnakes, as all three are similar in habits and habitats.

Dusky Pygmy Rattlesnake

(subspecies *barbouri*)

PHOTO #10

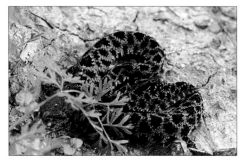

The dusky pygmy is the darkest of the three types of pygmy rattlers, being charcoal gray with black saddles down the middle of the back and smaller black spots on the sides. It also has reddish brown spots on the top of the back between the black saddles. The record length of the dusky pygmy is 32¹/₂ inches, the longest of the three subspecies, and they will also, on average, be larger than their two cousins. Still, most adults will be less than 2 feet in length.

Dusky pygmys range throughout peninsular Florida and northward into south Georgia, southern Alabama and southeast Mississippi where they intergrade with their northern cousins the Carolina and Western pygmys. In much of Florida, these little rattlers are quite common, especially in the Everglades region in the southern part of the state. Throughout the sunshine state, they frequently show up in lawns and gardens in rural areas where they pose a risk to pets, gardeners, and barefoot children. Bites to humans occur frequently in Florida and while not life threatening, they are quite painful and can cause permanent tissue damage, and in the case of an infant or very small toddler the bite of this snake would be cause for grave concern.

During the years I lived in Florida in the 1970s, I saw a great many of these diminutive rattlesnakes in a variety of habitats and locations throughout the state. In recent excursions to their haunts, they seem much less common. Sadly, this is not a surprising development given the massive changes wrought on the landscape of Florida over the last few decades.

Western Pygmy Rattlesnake

(subspecies *streckeri*)

PHOTO #11 (right) & 29

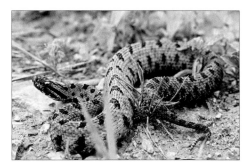

This race differs from the preceding two by being much browner in color. Like the other two subspecies, the characteristic dark saddles on the back are separated by smaller reddish brown spots, but the overall color between the blotches is much browner. See photos. This is the most wide-ranging member of the pygmy rattlesnake group, being found from Mississippi westward to eastern Texas, and from the gulf coast north to the Missouri Ozarks and western Kentucky. Oddly, it is absent from a broad swath along the Mississippi River valley (see range map).

Western pygmys are the smallest of the three subspecies, with a record length of only 25 inches. Most are fully grown at 18 inches. The largest individual I have seen measured just a bit over 23 inches and came from the Land Between the Lakes National Recreation Area in western Kentucky. Over the years I have seen a half-dozen specimens from this area, a paltry amount given the number of hours I have spent trekking through this 600,000-acre woodland. While most of those I have seen here were in typically moist woodland near water, I did find one high on a ridge top in xeric (dry) woodland. I have also seen a few from the Ozarks region of northern Arkansas where I found them in cedar glades in the vicinity of streams.

From discussions with local residents there, I am inclined to conclude that they are more common here than in many areas of their range.

The eastern hognose snake is the non-venomous snake most often confused with this subspecies (see photo #78). A friend of mine who for years taught herpetology at Murray State University actually had a student bitten by a western pygmy rattlesnake when the student mistook it for a harmless hognose snake and picked it up! The mishap occurred during a field trip for a herpetology class. The student recovered completely and went on to receive a passing grade in the class despite his identification faux pas. For additional information, read the preceding account for this species.

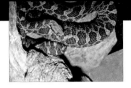

MASSASAUGA RATTLESNAKES
(Sistrurus catenatus)

The Massasaugas represent a large and heavy-bodied version of the pygmy rattlesnakes, occasionally reaching a length of just over 3 feet. Like their cousins the pygmy rattlers, massasaugas possess a fairly toxic venom, and their larger size equates to a larger dose of venom. Though many experts question their ability to kill a healthy adult, their bite often produces serious systemic reactions, and herpetologist Carl Ernst in his book *Venomous Reptiles of North America* states that deaths from massasauga bites have occurred. This species should be considered at least potentially deadly.

Though I have kept a number of these snakes in captivity over the years, I have never seen one in the wild (they are becoming increasingly rare), and I have thus relied heavily on previously published material in writing the accounts of the three subspecies found in the United States.

Wetlands are the prime habitat for these snakes in the eastern portions of their range and they are the most aquatic of all rattlesnakes. Their peculiar name was given to them by the Chippewa Indians. For more information, read the following accounts of the three subspecies and see the range map below.

Like the closely related pygmy rattlesnakes, the massasaugas are considered by experts to be evolutionarily intermediate between the genus *Agkistrodon* (copperheads and cottonmouths) and the genus *Crotalus* (true rattlesnakes). The respective ranges of the three subspecies appear below.

RANGE OF THE MASSASSAUGA IN THE UNITED STATES

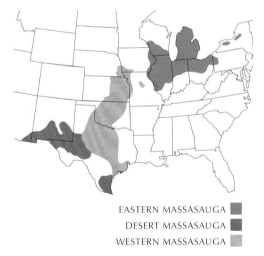

EASTERN MASSASAUGA ■
DESERT MASSASAUGA ■
WESTERN MASSASAUGA ■

Eastern Massasauga
(subspecies *catenatus*)

PHOTO #21 (right) & 28

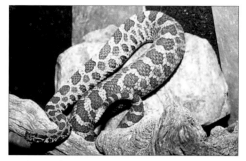

The eastern massasauga is the darkest of the three subspecies of the massasauga, being charcoal gray to smoky gray with darker gray or black blotches on the back. There are also small dark spots on the sides that match the dorsal blotches in color. In many respects this snake closely resembles its smaller cousin, the dusky pygmy rattlesnake, but lacks the small reddish brown spots between the dark dorsal blotches that characterize the pygmy rattlers. I have seen photos of individuals from Ontario, Canada, that were russet brown with dark gray blotches.

This eastern race is also the largest of its species, reaching a record length of 39 1/2 inches, though most average about 2 to 2 1/2 feet as adults. As with all American pit vipers, the 8- to 9-inch-long young are born alive, and except for being more vividly patterned are miniature replicas of the adults. The litter size may exceed a dozen in the case of a large, mature female.

This is one of the northernmost ranging venomous snakes in America, found as far north as southern Ontario in Canada. They are sometimes called "swamp rattlers," an appropriate name since they are the most aquatic of all rattlesnakes. Their preferred habitat is bogs and marshes and they have even been known to hibernate in crawfish burrows. This subspecies ranges throughout what was formerly mostly tall grass prairie, though they may also be found in woodlands. The disappearance of the tall grass prairies and associated draining of bogs and marshes as man converted the land to agricultural uses has greatly diminished the habitat for this subspecies and today they occur only in sporadic populations from western Pennsylvania across northern Ohio, Indiana, and Illinois to eastern Iowa and northeastern Missouri. They also range northward into Wisconsin and through Michigan into southern Ontario. A disjunct population occurs in New York.

Due to their increasing scarcity, these snakes are now protected by law in many places. According to John Levell in his book *A Field Guide to Reptiles and Amphibians and the Law*, they are listed as endangered in Illinois, Pennsylvania, Iowa, Wisconsin, and Missouri. Indiana considers them a threatened species. In Michigan and Minnesota they are currently listed as a species of special concern. Christiansen and Bailey in *The Snakes of Iowa* reported that in Iowa, "The remaining populations are now centered in three state-managed marshes." In Illinois they are found in only a few widely scattered and isolated populations where remnants of their original habitat remain. Phillips, Brandon, and Moll in *Reptiles and Amphibians of Illinois* state that these snakes were "Formerly common over the northern two thirds of the state, prior to the drainage of prairie marshes and intensive agriculture. Once known from 24 widely scattered relict populations, now thought to occur at only 6-8." Oldfield and Moriarty in *Amphibians and Reptiles Native to Minnesota* report that they occur in only two counties in that state. Their food consists mostly of mice and voles, but they have also been known to eat other snakes, frogs, and lizards.

Western Massasauga

(subspecies *tergiminus*)

PHOTO #32

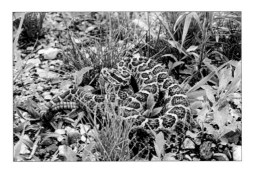

This subspecies differs from the eastern massasauga chiefly in color, being paler. Most are smoky gray with dark brown blotches as opposed to charcoal gray with black blotches. The record length of $34^3/4$ inches is slightly less than its eastern counterpart.

This is a snake of the central and southern plains. Most of its range is contained in Kansas, Oklahoma, and Texas, but it is also found in southeast Nebraska, extreme southwestern Iowa, and a tiny area of northwestern Missouri. It is much more common than its eastern relative, and was once quite abundant in select localities, though its numbers have diminished in recent times due mainly to the loss of prairie habitat to agriculture. Western massasaugas reportedly favor prairie bogs and marshes as habitat, though they may also be found in rocky outcrops in drier areas. In the southern plains where the summer sun can be unrelenting, they are primarily nocturnal animals, almost never seen during the day. Among the items listed as food for this subspecies are mice, lizards, small snakes, amphibians, and shrews.

These snakes often exhibit a peculiar behavior known as "gaping," in which the mouth is held at least partially open. This behavior is known to regularly occur in only one other venomous snake species in North America, the cottonmouth. Unlike cottonmouths that gape as part of a "threat display," the gaping of the western massasauga appears to be unrelated to any threat. In fact, a specimen from Kansas kept in captivity by the author for many years would gape only when undisturbed, and would often sit for hours in its cage with its mouth half opened. The author has not been able to find any explanation for this strange behavior in the reference material available on this snake.

Desert Massasauga
(subspecies *edwardsi*)
PHOTO #40

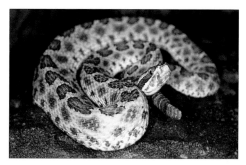

A still smaller and paler version of massasauga, this subspecies reaches a maximum length of only 21 inches. The belly of this race lacks the dark mottling, a characteristic that in itself distinguishes it from the other two massasaugas, both of whom have belly patterns consisting of a mottled gray.

This is a dwarf desert subspecies, being found mostly in desert grasslands in western Texas, southern New Mexico, and extreme southeastern Arizona. A disjunct population can also be found south of the Rio Grande in Mexico. It is the least abundant of its species, being rarely encountered and then usually at night, as it is unable to withstand the searing day-time heat of its Chihuahuan Desert habitat. During the day, it often takes refuge in burrows of small mammals like the kangaroo rat. Throughout its range it occurs only in sporadic localities of undisturbed desert grassland, and is curiously absent from some areas of apparently ideal habitat. It is considered rare throughout its range and is protected in Arizona. Desert massasaugas are known to feed on mice and lizards.

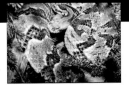

TIMBER AND CANEBRAKE RATTLESNAKES
(Crotalus horridus)

There are two subspecies of this snake recognized by the author, though many experts recognize only one, considering the canebrake to be merely a geographic variant of the timber. Other experts suggest that there may be as many as three subspecies.

This species is the most wide-spread rattlesnake in the eastern United States. Its range encompasses most of the eastern half of the nation from the central plains eastward, except for the far northern areas of the country. It is declining in many of the more populous areas, especially in the Northeast, and is today only locally abundant in many areas where it was once a common reptile. As with many wide-ranging species, considerable variation exists within the species and much of this variation relates directly to geographic locality.

Throughout much of their range, the timber and canebrake exhibit characteristics that are intermediate between the "true" timber and "true"canebrake forms. These intermediate forms are properly termed "intergrades" (see photo #24 for an example of a typical timber/canebrake intergrade). Due to the great variation exhibited by this species and the gradual melding of characters over a wide geographic area, some controversy exists

among herpetologists as to whether or not the timber and canebrake constitute two valid subspecies. I am convinced that they do and treat them accordingly in this book. The range map for the two subspecies appears below, and detailed information on the natural history of both races follows on subsequent pages.

RANGE OF THE TIMBER & CANEBRAKE RATTLESNAKES IN THE UNITED STATES

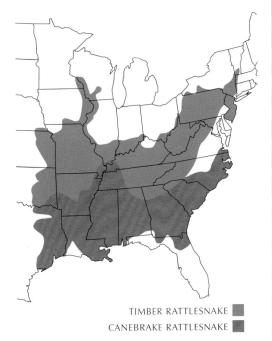

TIMBER RATTLESNAKE ▇
CANEBRAKE RATTLESNAKE ▇

Timber Rattlesnake

(subspecies *horridus*)

PHOTO #22, 23 (right), 24 & 30

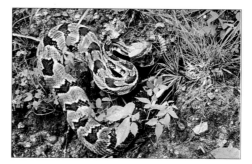

The name "timber rattlesnake" is highly appropriate as these animals live only in forests and woodlands. They are most abundant in the Appalachian Mountains but range through most of the eastern deciduous forest (see range map on page 107). Rugged, heavily wooded areas with rocky outcroppings are their favorite haunts. In the western portions of their range, where the deciduous forests begin to give way to prairie, they may be found locally in ravines and other wooded areas.

In the densely populated northeastern United States they have declined dramatically in recent years. The states of Vermont, New Hampshire, Massachusetts, Connecticut, New Jersey, Virginia, and Ohio all list the timber rattlesnake as an endangered species and it is considered threatened in New York, Indiana, and Illinois and protected in Rhode Island. Minnesota lists them as a species of special concern. They still exist in healthy numbers in much of the southern Appalachians and the Ozarks, and, in fact, they may be locally common in any area of their range where suitable habitat exists that is sufficiently remote from human activities.

The alarming reduction in timber rattlesnake populations is mostly attributable to habitat loss; but the propensity to hibernate in communal dens has also been a factor. In many of the northernmost areas of this snake's range, it is necessary for all reptiles to spend the winter deep underground below the depth where freezing temperatures penetrate earth. In New England or the upper Mississippi valley this may mean a depth of several feet. Finding places that allow easy access to suitable hibernacula can be a challenge, and thus where such places do exist, they may be used by dozens or even hundreds of snakes. Field studies have shown that snakes can imprint to a particular hibernating area, and the same winter den may be used for generations. When such a den is discovered by humans, it is vulnerable to exploitation. Snake collectors, hide hunters, or those who consider the only good rattlesnake a dead one have decimated den after den. In addition, many such places have been destroyed by land developers.

Another factor contributing to the decline of this and many other reptile species are highways. Countless thousands of snakes are killed annually while attempting to cross roadways, and a busy interstate acts as an impossible barrier to such slow-moving creatures. In addition to killing many snakes outright, a four-lane highway can fragment populations, preventing the dispersal of the gene pool. In the Shawnee National Forest in southern Illinois the U.S. Forest Service closes select roads through the forest during periods of migration to and from hibernating dens, an insightful conservation practice that is being utilized by too few state and federal agencies. Unfortunately, such practices are not possible for major highways and interstates. One solution is to use low, small mesh fences that funnel migrating snakes into small tunnels beneath the road, but this is almost never practiced by road builders.

Despite its increasing scarcity, the timber rattlesnake remains the rattlesnake most likely to be encountered by most outdoor enthusiasts in America. Fortunately, it is a snake that is not prone to strike unless seriously provoked. Most specimens in the wild will remain quiet and motionless when approached, only rattling and striking if trod upon or otherwise molested. Timbers can be dangerous snakes however! Their venom is quite toxic and large individuals are more than capable of delivering a dose that could be lethal to a human, and recorded deaths from their bite are numerous.

Timber rattlers from the southern Appalachian Mountains and Ozarks region may reach 6 feet in length (record 6 feet 2 inches). By contrast, specimens from New England rarely exceed 4 feet, and the book *Amphibians and Reptiles Native to Minnesota* by Oldfield and Moriarty gives a record length of 4 feet 5 inches for that state.

In color and pattern, the timber rattler is a highly variable snake, so much so that an attempt at a written description would be laborious for both author and reader. Thus, the reader is advised to look at the photos of the various color phases (Photos #22, 23, 24 & 30). Most individuals exhibit a dorsal pattern of dark chevron-shaped bands across the back, and the tail is jet black. In the

Appalachian Mountains and the Northeast, an almost jet-black color phase occurs, along with a sulfur yellow phase and almost any shade of yellowish, brownish, or grayish in between. All the lighter color phases show evidence of the dark chevrons across the back, and these markings are usually discernible on all but the darkest of the dark phase specimens.

The primary foods of the timber rattlesnake are small mammals, with chipmunks and squirrels being the primary prey for adults. They also prey heavily on deer mice, voles, and other small rodents that are the mainstay of the diet for the smaller young snakes. Birds and bird eggs are also eaten but do not constitute a significant portion of their diet. In at least some areas there seems to be a direct correlation between the eastern chipmunk and the timber rattlesnake, with rattlers being found in areas where chipmunks are common, and absent from those areas where there are no chipmunks (personal observation).

In hunting and feeding tactics, these snakes are ambush predators, preferring to lie in a motionless coil near a game trail or burrow entrance. Numerous reptile experts have reported the habit these snakes have of using fallen logs as ambush sites, a logical ploy since fallen logs are regularly traveled by both squirrels and chipmunks when foraging on the forest floor. This also accounts for the time-honored warning to hikers and hunters about snakebite avoidance, i.e., "don't step across a log, step up on it first and look on the other side." This is good advice but probably moot since the cryptic nature of this snake's color pattern usually renders it invisible to the average human, even when a few feet away. The difficulty in seeing these snakes in their natural habitat is obvious to those of us who have actively searched for them in the wooded hollows where they make their home. This point was dramatically illustrated in an instance related to the author by John McGregor, a well-known and highly respected biologist from Kentucky, who while accompanying another researcher seeking a wild timber with an implanted radio transmitter had great difficulty locating the snake even after being led by the transmitter to within a few feet of its location!

Young timber rattlers are born in late summer or early fall and resemble miniature adults and average about 11 inches in length. The litter size is usually around eight to 10, though large, well-fed females may produce twice as many young. Litter sizes are smaller in the northern populations, and females are slower to reach sexual maturity due to a shorter growing season (some may not breed until age seven or eight).

Additionally, the shorter summers give females less time to replenish the stored fat needed for successful embryo development, and females in the North are able to produce litters only every third or fourth year, while females living farther south can produce a litter every other year. This low reproductive rate, coupled with the human disturbance factors discussed earlier, adds up to a grim outlook for this subspecies in the Northeast. One saving grace that this rattlesnake shares with many other pit vipers is its longevity, some may live as much as 30 years.

Adult timber rattlesnakes have few enemies other than man. They may be preyed upon by the usual snake-eating carnivores (opossums, hawks, owls, kingsnakes), and sometimes even normally docile herbivores may kill rattlers in defense. Lawrence Klauber's classic book *Rattlesnakes: Their Habits, Life Histories, and Influence on Mankind* states that deer have been known to stomp rattlesnakes to death. Hogs are known to kill and eat all kinds of snakes, and populations of feral hogs in the southern Appalachians and Great Smoky Mountains may have a serious impact on timber rattlesnake populations.

Most of the wild timbers seen by the author were from Kentucky, Tennessee, and southern Illinois. The only examples I have seen from Kentucky that I would call good examples of the timber rattlesnake came from Pine Mountain and Black Mountain in the southeastern part of the state. Throughout much of the rest of Kentucky, specimens show some characters of intergradation with the southern canebrake rattler.

Canebrake Rattlesnake

(subspecies *atricaudatus*)

PHOTO #12 (right) & 13

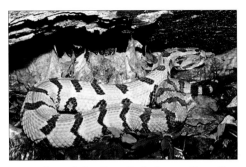

The canebrake rattlesnake is a southern, more lowland form of the timber rattlesnake. Unlike the upland loving timber, the canebrake can be found in low, wet woodlands and swamps of the coastal plain. In most other respects, it mimics the natural history of the timber rattler and the reader is referred to the account of the timber rattler on the preceding pages for data on food, reproduction, etc. In color and pattern it tends toward hues of pink and purple with the chevron-shaped crossbands always pronounced. There is also a broad orange to reddish stripe down the center of the back (see photo #12). The record length of this subspecies is 6 feet 2¹/2 inches, essentially the same as the record length for its cousin the timber rattler, but overall canebrakes will average larger, with 5-footers not uncommon among adult males. Females rarely exceed 4 feet.

Like many snakes, the canebrake exhibits a large degree of geographic variation. Individuals from the lower coastal plain of the southeastern United States are good examples of this subspecies, but farther north they begin to show evidence of intergradation with their northern cousin, the timber rattler. The zone of intergradation between the northern timber and the southern canebrake is so broad that there are probably at least as many individuals that could be characterized as intergrades as there are specimens that would be considered good examples of the "true" timber or "true" canebrake.

These intergrade populations show what biologists call a "clinal variation." In the case of the timber/canebrake rattlers, the "cline" is basically north to south. The farther north you are, the more the population resembles the northern subspecies (timber), and the farther south, the more the population resembles the southern race (canebrake). In reality, the clinal variation of the two snakes may be more related to elevation than to compass direction, with canebrakes being snakes of the low coastal plain and timbers occupying the higher ground farther inland. However, many intergrade populations of the canebrake rattlesnake occupy habitats similar to that of the timber rattlesnake, i.e., upland woods and wooded ridges.

All these factors tend to lend strong credence to the argument presented by many herpetologists that the two snakes should be considered as a single species. However, if you compare examples of the timber from the Appalachians (photo #22) with the canebrake from northern Florida (photo #12), you obviously are looking at two very different snakes. Studies of snake venoms have also shown evidence of physiological differences, namely the more potent aspect of the venom of the canebrake due to a higher amount of neurotoxins. I personally have no especially strong feelings regarding the taxonomic status of *Crotalus horridus*; some naturalists are "groupers", and some are "splitters." On this issue I come down on the side of the splitters.

I do have a strong opinion regarding the potential threat the canebrake represents to victims of its bite. In 1978, I was bitten on the left hand by a 4-foot canebrake that embedded both fangs into two fingers. The snake had just been handled at the time and was thoroughly aroused. The strike terminated in a strong bite with two "pumps" of the venom glands. Within 15 minutes I began to go into shock and in 30 minutes was unable to stand or even sit upright. Arriving at the emergency room of a local hospital at about 45 minutes post bite, I was lapsing in and out of consciousness and my blood pressure was undetectable. A massive infusion of intravenous fluids, vasoconstrictive drugs and 13 vials of antivenin (all that was available) finally neutralized the activity of the venom. The symptoms I experienced prior to losing consciousness for a period of hours included tingling in the legs, face, and tongue; vomiting, diarrhea, diaphoresis, and hypovolemic shock. Many experts on snakebite consider canebrakes of the lower coastal plain to be among our most dangerous snakes. I tend to agree.

Near my home in western Kentucky, the 600-square-mile Land Between the Lakes National Recreation Area (administered by the U.S. Forest Service) provides abundant habitat for a healthy population of timber/canebrake intergrades, and may soon become a "last stand" habitat for these diminishing animals in western Kentucky. In western Tennessee, they are also becoming a rare animal. In the Deep South, they seem to be faring somewhat better; and on one recent snake hunting expedition, conducted in the spring of 2002, four hunters collected a remarkable 17 canebrakes in one day's hunting in southern Georgia. The author has found these snakes to be fairly common still in the Osceola National Forest in northernmost Florida, an area that consists mostly of mesic pine woodlands and palmetto, interspersed with a great deal of permanent wetlands. In the lower coastal plain regions of southern Mississippi, Alabama, Georgia, and northern Florida, the canebrake rattlesnake is found sympatrically with the eastern diamondback rattlesnake. Where the ranges of the two snakes overlap, they are not usually found together. The book *The Reptiles and Amphibians of Alabama* by Robert Mount states that in Alabama "the diamondback is usually found in relatively dry, sandy situations, whereas the timber (canebrake) rattler is restricted mostly to swampy areas and floodplains." However, the author is aware of one instance where both the canebrake and diamondback were found sheltering beneath the same piece of tin in northern Florida, and on very rare occasions rattlesnakes have been found that possessed an unusual color and pattern that could only have resulted from the hybridization of the two species.

Eastern Diamondback Rattlesnake

(Crotalus adamanteus)

PHOTO #14 (right), 15 & 16

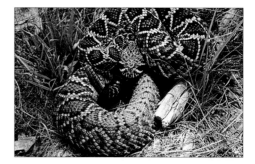

Compared with the most deadly known species of poisonous snakes of the world, the eastern diamondback ranks high. Its huge fangs and enormous venom glands represent the maximum degree of deadliness attained by the viperine serpents." Those words were written in 1936 by one of America's giants in the field of herpetology, Raymond Ditmars, and published in his classic work *The Reptiles of North America.* The respect he showed for this snake is well deserved. Large specimens may have fangs up to 1¹/₂ inches in length and it possess large amounts of highly toxic venom. It is hard to overstate the gravity of a bite by this snake and prior to the advent of antivenin and advanced treatment procedures, a very significant percentage of its victims died.

The record length of 8 feet, 3 inches was recorded by the above mentioned author over 50 years ago and it remains as the world record rattlesnake. The largest wild specimen ever examined by the author measured 6 feet 4 inches and weighed 13¹/₂ pounds. (See photo #16) In the decade of the 1970s, while working in Florida with herpetologist Ross Allen, the author saw many specimens in excess of 5 feet and several that exceeded 6 feet. Ross Allen himself over the 50-odd years in the snake business saw hundreds of thousands of these impressive serpents; the largest individual caught in the wild measured 7 feet 3 inches. During this period a cash reward for any rattlesnake of 8 feet was never collected, and some experts have questioned the validity of the 8-foot-3-inch specimen recorded by Ditmars in 1936. Today the species is in decline throughout its range and it is doubtful indeed that we shall ever see another 8-footer from the wild. There have been, however, a few well-fed captive raised specimens that have easily exceeded 7 feet. This fact, coupled with the impeccable reputation of Mr. Ditmars as a serious herpetologist, leads this author to believe in the validity of Mr. Ditmars' specimen.

The eastern diamondback is a snake of the southeastern United States and ranges along the lower coastal plain from

RANGE OF THE EASTERN DIAMONDBACK RATTLESNAKE IN THE UNITED STATES

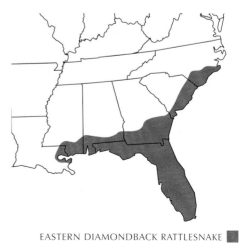

EASTERN DIAMONDBACK RATTLESNAKE ■

southeastern North Carolina to lower Mississippi, including all of Florida and many offshore islands (see range map). The favorite food of the adults is rabbits, and a fully grown snake can easily swallow a grown cottontail. In coastal areas and salt marshes, the smaller marsh rabbit can be quite plentiful and provide a stable food source. They also prey heavily on the native rodent the rice rat. Squirrels and other small mammals are eaten along with a few ground-nesting birds.

These snakes occupy nearly all types of habitats within their range except for large expanses of swamp, being most common in pine savannahs and scrub oak habitats where they often associate with the gopher tortoise, using the tortoise burrows as a retreat from cold snaps or searing summer heat. They may also be found in pine flatwoods and are frequently along the edges of salt marshes.

While employed at the Ross Allen Reptile Institute and later at the St. Augustine Alligator Farm during the 1970s, I had the occasion to see many thousands of specimens of these magnificent serpents. The most unusual was a 3-foot specimen collected in 1972 near Whigham, Georgia, by a local resident. This snake was a uniform brown with a faint black mid-dorsal stripe. This unique specimen resided at the Ross Allen Reptile Institute in Silver Springs for several years and though it never fed on its own, it was kept alive by force-feeding. It never seemed to grow and sadly died while in my care. It is now in the preserved collection of the Florida State Museum in Gainesville. Interestingly, it is not the only such specimen on record. In a 1959 issue of *Florida Naturalist* magazine, there is a photograph of an eastern diamondback identical to this specimen.

Most of the author's personal experiences with these impressive reptiles in the wild have occurred in the Ocala National Forest in central Florida where thirty years ago they were not uncommon. For a snake hunter the experience of encountering a massive eastern diamondback is memorable. I vividly recall one such experience that happened while I was employed by the St. Augustine Alligator Farm on Florida's east coast. A young boy came by to tell us about a huge rattlesnake he had found coiled beneath a clump of palmetto on the edge of a nearby salt marsh. When the boy, Ross Allen and myself returned to the scene, the boy led us to the exact patch of palmettos where the snake had been sighted. The three of us searched for fully 10 minutes before the youngster once again located the snake, which had moved about ten feet and was quietly coiled beneath another clump of saw palmetto. I had nearly stepped on the snake several times! Even after seeing it, I could turn my gaze away and have difficulty locating it again. Such is the effectiveness of this animal's cryptic coloration. The snake was a real whopper, just under six feet in length and very fat. It could have bitten any one of us several times as we searched for it, but instead relied for defense on its exquisite camouflage. This behavior is typical for the species, as they rarely rattle unless provoked.

An even more convincing example of their reluctance to bite is illustrated by a maneuver that was taught to me by the late Ross Allen, who was both an accomplished herpetologist and inveterate showman. Standing directly in front of a coiled and rattling snake, it is possible to lean forward with the arm extended, and coming in from directly above actually touch the snake on the top of the head without (usually) eliciting a strike. It is with some chagrin that I admit to having performed this risky maneuver a number of times and can only claim as a defense the foolhardy brashness of youth. For the benefit of any young readers let me state unequivocally that such bravado is how most snakebites occur, and in the case of a snake like the eastern diamondback, it is a darn good way to get yourself killed!

Despite its often-serene nature, when aroused this snake can be quite intimidating. Raising the head and neck slightly, they will rattle loudly and follow an adversary's every movement, usually not striking until the target is within range. Rarely, when really fighting for their life, these snakes will employ another defense, which is to position the tail so that the cloaca is aimed in the direction of the attacker and squirt musk from glands at the base of the tail. The musk is quite pungent and its unpleasant odor is complemented by the fact that it burns the eyes and mucous membranes. I have had rattlesnakes spray this musk into my face from a distance of 6 feet, and have witnessed this on several occasions by many species of rattlesnake.

It is fortunate that these formidable snakes are not easily provoked, for they are among the world's most dangerous serpents. I knew several people who worked at the Ross Allen Reptile Institute who survived bites and many, including

Ross Allen, bore the scars of deformed or missing digits as a result. I was bitten once in the base of the thumb by a large specimen; but my guardian angel was on duty that day and it proved to be a minimal injection that did not require treatment, although the lymph nodes in the armpit remained swollen and sore for several days after.

It is impossible for me to write about the eastern diamondback without saying more about Mr. E. Ross Allen, who probably saw more of these snakes than anyone who ever lived. Today, younger herpetologists deride the practices he condoned, such as attending rattlesnake roundups to purchase snakes for use in venom production that were ultimately slaughtered for their skins. While such practices today are rightly condemned, when viewed in a historical context it is much easier to understand.

The Ross Allen Reptile Institute was founded when much of Florida was a wild and unspoiled wilderness and some of the native reptile fauna posed a real threat to the human inhabitants. Men like Allen were hailed for their work in reducing the abundant populations of venomous reptiles, as well as for their ability to educate and inform a population that was terribly ignorant of the role of wildlife in the local ecology. Snakes and Alligators were vermin to most, but Allen saw them as a resource. To his credit, with the passage of time, he became more and more of a conservationist, and his lifelong dedication to informing and educating the public about wildlife had, in the end, a positive impact that cannot be overstated.

Western Diamondback Rattlesnake

(Crotalus atrox)

PHOTO #34 (right) & 38

This wide-ranging rattlesnake occurs from west-central Arkansas westward across the south-western United States to extreme southeastern California. Its range includes most of the southern half of Oklahoma, nearly all of Texas, except the forested easternmost third of the state, and most of southern New Mexico and Arizona. It also ranges across much of northern Mexico (except Baja). See range map for exact range.

The western diamondback is primarily a desert and arid grassland animal, but they do range eastward into the westernmost edge of the deciduous forests in eastern Oklahoma and west-central Arkansas. This species is a habitat generalist, being found in all types of habi-

RANGE OF THE WESTERN DIAMONDBACK RATTLESNAKE IN THE UNITED STATES

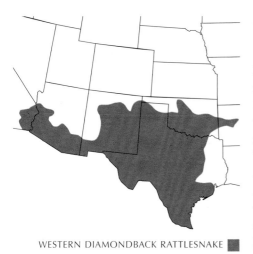

WESTERN DIAMONDBACK RATTLESNAKE ■

tats within its range except for moist environments. It is most common in dry scrub, desert, and rocky habitats and ranges from sea level to an elevation of about 7,000 feet. In addition to being wide ranging, they are also perhaps the most numerous large rattlesnake in America, being very common in many areas of its range.

Like its southeastern counterpart, (eastern diamondback), the western diamondback is a large and highly dangerous snake. In size, they average every bit as large as the eastern diamondback, though the record is somewhat less at 7 feet 8 inches. And though smaller at birth than the eastern diamondback, experiments with captive breeding seem to indicate that the western diamondback may possess the genetic material to attain a greater size. This fact was revealed by one wealthy individual who indulged himself for some time in an attempt to rear an 8-foot rattlesnake. In his experiments, the western diamondbacks consistently outgrew the easterns, growing faster and most attaining a larger size. Though the goal of an 8-footer was never achieved, the experiment is legendary among herpetologists and zookeepers for the massive snakes it did produce, some of which exceeded 7$^1/_2$ feet in length and had a girth the size of a man's thigh!

While most wild western diamondbacks are 4 to 5 feet as adults, a number of wild caught 7-footers have been recorded. The population in extreme southeastern Texas along the lower Rio Grande is where most of the really big wild snakes have been found, while farther west in the less productive desert regions most individuals are fully grown at about 4 to 4¹/₂ feet.

These snakes are highly irritable and perhaps quicker to strike than any other snake in America. They are irascible creatures that more often than not instantly react to provocation by whipping into a high coil, rattling incessantly and striking repeatedly at anything that comes near. While their venom is not as toxic as the eastern diamondback's, or for that matter many other rattlesnake's, they are still credited with more snakebite deaths than any other snake in America. This may be due in part to the fact that many bites by this species occur on remote rangelands and ranches where medical help may be hours away. However, its reputation as the snake that kills the most may be misleading, since many of the deaths attributed to this species over the years may well have been caused by a smaller, but much more deadly look-alike, the Mojave rattlesnake, which inhabits much of the same range (see photo #39).

Most victims of the western diamondback do survive, with the mortality rate estimated to be about one in ten. Still, even though the western diamondback's venom is relatively weak when compared to many other rattlers, its strike is capable of injecting a larger dose than any other rattlesnake, and its

long fangs (up to 1¹/₄ inches) can deliver the venom deep into muscle where it is instantly absorbed. All these factors—large fangs and venom glands, wide range and abundance, and a thoroughly pugnacious attitude—have earned this snake its well-deserved reputation as a highly dangerous reptile.

The author has kept a number of these snakes in captivity over the years and has seen scores of specimens in the wild, and while the rare individual may exhibit a more docile nature, the vast majority remained quick to strike even after long periods in captivity. In color and pattern, these snakes exhibit the classic diamond-shaped blotches down the entire length of the body; in overall color it may be light gray, dark gray, brownish, or rarely even reddish (see photos #34 and 38). They are often called "coontail" rattlers because of the pronounced black and white rings present on the tail. This trait is shared with the smaller Mojave rattlesnake, with which the western diamondback is often confused. Close examination of the tails of the two species will reveal that on the Mojave rattler the white bands are much wider, while on the western diamondback the white and black bands are equal in width.

These snakes are primarily crepuscular and nocturnal during warmer months, but may be seen abroad at midday during the early spring and fall. In the Sonoran Desert region of Arizona, they seem most common along dry washes and creek beds where vegetation is more abundant, and in the Chihuahuan Deserts of west Texas and New Mexico they are commonly seen on rural roads in a wide variety of habitats. Near Big Bend National Park in extreme west Texas, it is sometimes possible to see more than a dozen individuals in a few hours of "road cruising" under ideal conditions.

Adults feed on a wide variety of small mammals, with rodents, birds, cottontails, and even jackrabbits being consumed. The young are identical in appearance to adults and average about 10 to 11 inches in length. The litter size can be quite large, up to two dozen, and some females may be capable of producing a litter annually, which may account in part for their abundance.

The author's most memorable experience with this species occurred in the Sonoran Desert of Arizona near the Mexican border. I encountered a 4-footer crossing a dirt road and as the snake was an exceptionally beautiful specimen, I decided to detain it momentarily for a photo and video session. I needed to move the snake to a suitable area for the task but to my dismay the snake hook that makes its permanent home in the

bed of my truck was nowhere to be found. Not to be denied, I searched around and finally found a 12-inch-long lug wrench with which I proceeded to attempt to scoop the snake into a container. To say that the terrified and thoroughly enraged rattler put up a spirited defense would be a gross understatement. After about five minutes of what can only be described as "combat," the fierce little diamondback was finally tired enough to allow himself to be boxed. I was accompanied at the time by a companion who was not a snake enthusiast and who found all the excitement to be almost more than he could bear! After waiting a decent interval to allow the enraged rattler to settle down, I placed the snake in a location nearby that was suitable for photography and began taking pictures. My completely unnerved companion remained in the truck as I accomplished the mission and then released the snake to resume his life among the harsh but enchanting landscape of cholla, ocotillo, and organ pipe cactus.

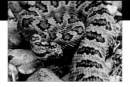

WESTERN RATTLESNAKE GROUP
(Crotalus viridis)

The common name western rattlesnake is very appropriate for this group of rattlesnakes comprising a total of eight subspecies. Together they give this species the widest range of any venomous snake in America. They can be found from Mexico to Canada and their collective ranges include the entire western half of the continental United States.

The western rattlesnakes occupy a variety of habitats from grassland to desert to high mountains. About the only habitat in the West where these snakes cannot be found is in the really hot deserts of lowest elevation. In virtually all other western habitats they may be found from sea level to an elevation of up to 10,000 feet, though they are rarely above 7,000 feet. The eight subspecies are differentiated based on color and pattern, and considerable variation exists between subspecies. All eight races are characterized by a pattern of rhomboid dorsal blotches that become ringlike on the tail. Some subspecies may migrate several miles each spring and fall to and from suitable hibernating areas, which are often in fissures of rock.

The primary prey of this species are small mammals, but the list of food items recorded includes lizards, amphibians, birds, and invertebrates. Below is a map depicting the range of the eight subspecies. Accounts of their natural histories follow on subsequent pages.

RANGE OF THE WESTERN RATTLESNAKE IN THE UNITED STATES

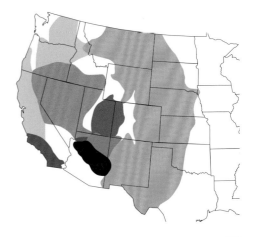

PRAIRIE RATTLESNAKE
HOPI RATTLESNAKE
MIDGET FADED RATTLESNAKE
GRAND CANYON RATTLESNAKE
GREAT BASIN RATTLESNAKE
ARIZONA BLACK RATTLESNAKE
NORTHERN PACIFIC RATTLESNAKE
SOUTHERN PACIFIC RATTLESNAKE

Prairie Rattlesnake

*(*subspecies *viridis)*

PHOTO #33, 55 (right) & 58

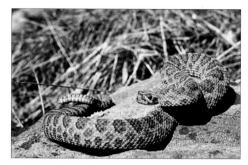

The Prairie Rattlesnake, as its name implies, is an animal mostly of the prairies and grasslands. Its range includes most of the mixed and short grass prairie regions from Canada to Mexico and it is America's most northerly ranging venomous snake, being found as far north as the high plains of Alberta and Saskatchewan in Canada. This subspecies also ranges up into mountainous areas along the eastern slope of the Rocky Mountains as high as 10,000 feet, but they are most common below 7,500 feet elevation. The scientific name *viridis* literally means green, and indeed most prairie rattlers have a greenish brown or greenish yellow tint, and some are decidedly light green with darker greenish brown blotches (see photos #33, #55, and #58). In size this is one of the larger of the viridis group, reaching a maximum (record) length of 4 feet. 10 inches.

The author has kept a number of prairie rattlesnakes in captivity and has observed in the wild several dozen individuals, mostly in western South Dakota and eastern Wyoming where they are still a fairly common snake, though less so than a few decades ago.

In the high northern plains they seem most common in the more rugged and eroded "badlands" habitats where rocky outcrops can be found. On flatter, more gently rolling prairie they are common around prairie dog towns where the numerous burrows provide a safe retreat from both the blazing summer sun and the bitter cold of the northern prairie.

This writer has also seen them in mountain canyons and pine forests in the Black Hills of South Dakota and the Big Horn Mountains of Wyoming. Their list of habitats includes virtually all biomes found within their range with the exception of low-lying desert. Though they may range well up into the mountains, they are much more common on foothill slopes and canyons, especially around areas of talus or rock outcrops.

This subspecies is well known in the northern plains for their communal hibernating dens, which may sometimes contain dozens (or in historical times hundreds) of snakes. The really large dens are now largely a thing of the past in most of the prairies' range, the result of years of persecution by man and changes wrought on the prairie by modern agricultural practices.

These rattlesnakes are in my experience more nervous in temperament than some others. Of those I have kept in captivity, most remained fairly quick to rattle and to strike even after considerable time in captivity. They are likewise more apt to rattle in the wild when approached by a large animal like a human. I remember an occasion when I encountered a 4-footer while climbing a steep ridge that rose out of the surrounding prairie in Carbon County, Wyoming. Upon hearing the unmistakable buzz of a rattlesnake some distance ahead and above, I hurried forward to investigate and covered a good 30 feet before finding the snake in a "high coil," thoroughly aroused and ready for defense. There was a strong crosswind so I am sure the snake had not detected me with olfactory senses, and as snakes have no tympanic membrane or external ear opening, it is certain he did not hear me. He may have detected the vibration of my footsteps but I tend to doubt his ability to do that at that distance; all of which leads me to believe that the snake was reacting to sight. The entire experience got me to thinking about the rattle of the rattlesnakes and how and why such a specialized structure came into being.

The widely held belief among biologists is that the rattle evolved as a means of warning large hoofed animals like bison to the presence of the snake beneath their feet, thereby preventing the snake from being trod upon. In this case, the snake certainly gave me an ample warning of its presence. Many other types of snakes, both harmless and venomous, will when threatened rapidly shake or vibrate the tip of their tail. Copperheads, cottonmouths, rat snakes, kingsnakes, and bullsnakes among others will exhibit this behavior. In addition to serving as notice of their presence, this tail vibrating also serves the important function of distracting an attacker's focus away from the vulnerable head to the less vulnerable tail, while the head is free to strike in defense. The rattle of the rattlesnakes undoubtedly developed as an extension of this serpentine behavior.

Prairie rattlers feed on a wide variety of small vertebrate prey including mice, voles, and gophers, as well as larger rodents like the prairie dog. In addition to a wide variety of small mammals, their list of food items also includes nestling birds, lizards, and amphibians. They are in turn preyed on by a variety of predators including other snakes, most notably yellow bellied racers, which will readily kill and eat the young. In a captive situation at Black Hills Reptile Gardens in South Dakota where large numbers of prairie rattlers were housed in an exposed pit with numerous bullsnakes and yellow bellied racers, I on two occasions observed racers kill and eat prairie rattlers. In one instance the rattlesnake was nearly as large as the racer that swallowed it. Racers are widespread and common throughout the range of the prairie rattlesnake and it is reasonable to assume they constitute a significant predation threat. Large buteo hawks like the ferruginous and red-tailed hawk, along with their larger cousin the golden eagle, are widespread throughout most of this snake range and all are confirmed rattlesnake eaters.

Like all pit vipers, prairie rattlesnakes are livebearers. The approximately 10-inch-long babies are usually born in the late summer or fall and number from two or three up to 15 or 20. Six to eight is an average litter.

Most of the author's personal experience with this snake came during a five-year professional relationship with the Black Hills Reptile Gardens just outside of Rapid City, South Dakota. This facility is a premier reptile exhibit. My association there not only increased my knowledge and understanding of rattlesnakes, but of reptiles in general.

Northern Pacific Rattlesnake

(subspecies *oreganus*)

PHOTO #63

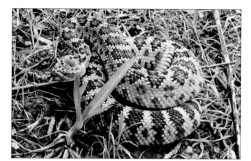

This race of the western rattlesnake occurs in eastern Washington, north-central Idaho, much of Oregon, and most of the northern two-thirds of California (see range map). It also ranges northward into Canada in a small area of British Columbia. Because of its presence in cooler, more northerly climates, the Northern Pacific rattler is more diurnal than many other rattlesnakes. Adults of this race typically reach a length of 3 to 3½ feet in length but the record length is a very respectable 5 feet 4 inches according to Carl Ernst in *Venomous Reptiles of North America.*

This snake is usually associated with dry grasslands and rocky areas. For instance, in the state of Washington it is absent from the rainy, sodden western slope of the Pacific ranges, preferring the drier, sunny areas farther inland where it can be fairly common. Andy Koukoulis, curator of reptiles for many years at the former Ross Allen Reptile Institute, reported to this author that decades ago this snake was often exceedingly common in many areas of Washington, so much so that he once caught 12 individuals in a single day's hunting on foot in a dry foothill canyon; and it is apparently still quite numerous in selected areas.

Its natural history is similar to that of its cousin the prairie rattlesnake discussed previously. Like the prairie rattler, this subspecies is renowned for its communal hibernating dens that can contain large numbers of snakes. Such dens are usually located in fissures of rock or in piles of talus. Small mammals are the primary prey but lizards, birds, and amphibians are also reportedly eaten. Its distinctive uniform tail bands help distinguish it from its very similar cousin, the more southerly ranging Southern Pacific rattlesnake.

The author's personal experience with this snake in the wild is limited to a few specimens kept in captivity. Thus, previously published material has been heavily relied upon in writing this account. An excellent source of further information on this subspecies can be found in the Seattle Audubon Society publication *Reptiles of Washington and Oregon.*

Southern Pacific Rattlesnake

(subspecies *helleri*)

PHOTO #62

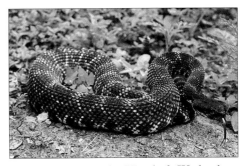

Very similar to the Northern Pacific rattlesnake discussed on the previous page, but the Southern Pacific rattler is overall darker in color, many specimens being almost black, and with the tail bands much less distinct. Young specimens are more vividly patterned, resembling somewhat the northern subspecies. This subspecies is so similar to the Arizona black rattlesnake (photo #49) that some experts have suggested that the range of the two races were once continuous, having been separated only recently in geological terms by the creation of desert expanses between southern California and the Mogollon Rim area of Arizona.**

The Southern Pacific rattlesnake is found throughout the western half of southern California exclusive of the Mojave Desert region and southward throughout Baja Norte, Mexico. They may be found in a variety of habitats, especially chaparral foothills.

The venom of this race of *viridis* is treacherously toxic. Even in the case of minimal envenomation, a serious drop in blood platelets can occur, even though other symptoms may not be pronounced. Such was the case in a bite to one of my reptile keepers at the Woods & Wetlands Wildlife Center in 1995. Though it was only a slight envenomation involving one fang on a fingertip and there was only moderate swelling reaching to the elbow, little discoloration and no necrosis, there was a progressive drop in blood platelets over a 48-hour period. Happily, the young man weathered the bite without incident and no antivenin was required.

This snake can reach a length of up to 4¹/₂ feet and it ranges throughout much of the highly populated southern California area. This coupled with their dangerously toxic venom make this subspecies perhaps the most threatening to man of the western rattlesnake group. In addition, they have been known to hybridize with the even more deadly Mojave rattlesnake in the Antelope valley of California. The predators and prey of this subspecies are probably not appreciably different from that given for the prairie and Northern Pacific rattlers.

** In the years since the original publication of this volume, DNA analysis has determined that the Southern Pacific and Arizona Black Rattlesnakes are, in fact, two distinct species.

Great Basin Rattlesnake
(subspecies *lutosus*)
PHOTO #61

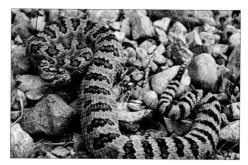

This subspecies ranges throughout the Great Basin Region, with most of its range comprising the greatest portion of the state of Nevada, but also being found in southern Idaho, south-central Oregon, eastern Utah, and extreme northwest Arizona. Throughout most of this large geographic area, it is the only venomous snake.

The color pattern of this snake consists of the series of rhomboid blotches on the back that characterize all races of the western rattlesnake. There is considerable variation within this subspecies, and the variation reflects the predominant colors of the habitat substrate, a common phenomenon among many western rattlesnakes. One of the most pronounced examples of the relationship between this snake's color and its environment was illustrated in a specimen I collected in Nye County, Nevada, near Lunar Crater. In that area for several square miles the desert floor is a creamy yellow sand littered with small pieces of black volcanic rock, presumably scattered across the landscape in an ancient explosion of great magnitude. The specimen I collected in this area was a large adult whose color and pattern perfectly replicated the substrate. Its color was the exact shade of creamy yellow as the sand, with solid black dorsal blotches that in size and shade mimicked the widespread black pebbles that littered the ground throughout the region. The color and pattern of this snake was so unique and striking that when I showed it to friends at the Black Hills Reptile Gardens in Rapid City, South Dakota, they insisted on having it and as far as I know, it resides there still.

In warmer months I have found these snakes to be not uncommonly seen at night on the lonely stretches that characterize many miles of roadway in the Great Basin Region. During the heat of the day they undoubtedly shelter underground. In many areas where they may be found the land is flat and lacks any canyons or rocky outcrops that provide shelter for so many desert species. The major plant component here is sagebrush, which I doubt would offer enough respite from the blistering heat of the Great Basin summer, and thus it is logical to assume that they spend their days in the numerous rodent burrows found here.

In size, this race is medium large, reaching a maximum length of about $4^{1}/_{2}$ feet. Like all larger members of its species, it is a dangerous snake that is capable of killing. The toxicity of its venom may vary in snakes from different geographical areas, and it has been known to intergrade with both the midget faded rattlesnake and the Grand Canyon rattlesnake where their respective ranges abut its own. Also, I have seen one individual from southeastern Oregon that was undoubtedly an intergrade with the Northern Pacific rattlesnake. The natural history of this race (prey, predators, etc.) is not significantly different from that of the prairie rattlesnake and the reader is referred to the account for that subspecies for further data.

Hopi Rattlesnake

(subspecies *nuntius*)

PHOTO #60

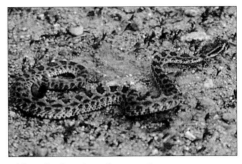

The Hopi rattlesnake is a smaller version of the prairie rattlesnake and whose basic biology is very similar to that subspecies. It differs in being smaller, averaging only about 2 feet in length (maximum 2 feet 4 inches), and in tending toward a more brownish coloration (often with a reddish tint). Their range is contained almost exclusively in the northeastern quadrant of Arizona within the ancestral lands of the Hopi Indians, who used these dangerously venomous serpents in a ritual that involved dancing around while holding the snake in either the hand or the mouth.

These little rattlers seem less common than other subspecies of *viridis*, and despite spending a day hiking and an evening road hunting within their territory (in preparation for writing this book), the author was unable to find one.

Grand Canyon Rattlesnake

(subspecies *abyssus*)

PHOTO #56

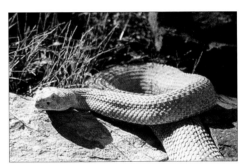

As their name implies, this race of the western rattlesnake is an inhabitant of Arizona's Grand Canyon Region. They are generally much more reddish in color than all other races of *viridis* and their pattern is much less distinct. The author has seen only two examples of this subspecies, one of which appears in this book. Both were in the collection of Jim Harrison of the Kentucky Reptile Zoo. Specimens from within the Grand Canyon are good examples of this race in its truest form, while around the canyon rim they show signs of intergradation with three other subspecies whose ranges surround the canyon (see range map). Thus, the range of the "true" Grand Canyon rattlesnake is quite small, and as a result they are protected by law in the state of Arizona.

The biology of this rare rattlesnake is currently being studied; it is assumed that their natural history is akin to that of the other races of western rattler. They are a moderate size rattler that can reach a maximum length of just over 3 feet.

Arizona Black Rattlesnake

(subspecies *cerberus*)

PHOTO #49

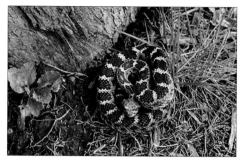

This is another appropriately named rattlesnake, as it is one of the very few truly black colored rattlers in America, and it is found mostly within Arizona. On the darkest specimens, the dorsal blotches that characterize all other subspecies of *viridis* may be obscured. Arizona blacks are highland animals, being found in chaparral and juniper foothills and mountain pine forests along the Mogollon Rim area of Arizona and exteme west-central New Mexico.

The Arizona black is very close in both appearance and habitat preference to the Southern Pacific rattlesnake and the two races may have once constituted a continuous population in an earlier time before the desertification of the southwestern United States. It is a small to medium size rattlesnake, averaging less than 3 feet in length and reaching a maximum of about $3^{1}/_{2}$ feet The biology of this race is assumed like that of other subspecies of *viridis*.*

Midget Faded Rattlesnake

(subspecies *concolor*)

PHOTO #59

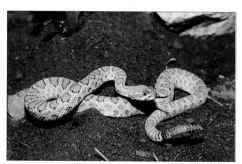

This is the smallest race of the western rattler group, and adults are fully grown at less than 2 feet. The largest recorded specimen the author could find in the literature reviewed was given as $25^{1}/_{2}$ inches. Despite their small size, they are dangerous snakes, with venom potency as much as 10 to 30 times greater than other members of their species.

They can be described as a dwarfed, bleached-out version of the prairie rattler, with the dorsal blotches sometimes barely discernible. Their overall coloration is very pale cream, tan, or brownish yellow. They are found in western Colorado and eastern Utah, but range barely up into Wyoming along the Green River in Sweetwater County.

Not much is known about these rattlesnakes, and they seem to be uncommon. Baxter and Stone in *Amphibians and Reptiles of Wyoming* report they are "found in rocky outcroppings in the sagebrush desert."

* In the years since the original publication of this volume, DNA analysis has determined that the Southern Pacific and Arizona Black Rattlesnakes are, in fact, two distinct species.

Mojave Rattlesnake
(Crotalus scutulatus)
PHOTO #39

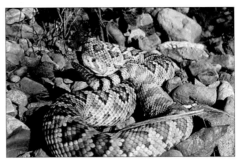

This is arguably America's most dangerous snake species. Its venom, drop for drop, can be many times more toxic than that of the western diamondback, which is the snake credited with more snakebite deaths than any other United States snake. Similar in appearance to the western diamondback and occupying many of the same desert regions of the Southwest, it can reasonably be assumed that at least some of the snakebite deaths attributed to the western diamondback over the years were actually bites inflicted by the Mojave rattler. The potency of this snake's venom has been shown to vary from one geographic area to another; thus, some Mojaves are much more dangerous than others. Those that possess the powerful nerve toxin now known as "mojave toxin" are the ones that are most lethal. In respect to the way the "Mojave toxin" kills by blocking nerve impulses, this snake's venom is similar to the cobra's and the American coral snake.

In comparison to the western diamondback, the Mojave is a smaller species, averaging about 3 feet in length, though they can reach a respectable size of over 4 feet. The record length is 51 inches.

This snake's range in the United States includes westernmost Texas, extreme southern New Mexico, much of Arizona, the southern tip of Nevada, and the Mojave Desert region of California (see range map). They are much more widespread south of the border in Mexico where at least one other subspecies occurs. Unlike many other southwestern rattlesnakes, which may range high up into mountainous areas, the Mojave rattler is an animal of the desert, being found at lower elevations in foothills and desert flats. Their name comes from the fact that the first specimens described to science were from the Mojave Desert, though they are also found in two other desert regions, the Chihuahuan and Sonoran Deserts.

In some parts of its range in California, the Mojave can be a fairly common snake, but in most areas it is

RANGE OF THE MOJAVE RATTLESNAKE IN THE UNITED STATES

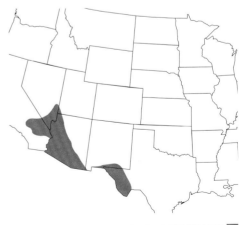

MOJAVE RATTLESNAKE ■

less abundant than the similar western diamondback. Distinguishing these two can be done by comparing the "coon tail" patterns seen on both snakes. In the western diamondback's "coon tail" pattern, the black rings are about equal in width to the alternating white rings, while in the Mojave rattler, the black rings are noticeably narrower than the white rings. Another similar rattlesnake species, the prairie rattlesnake, also occurs within parts of the Mojave's range (west Texas mostly). Prairie rattlers can be differentiated from the Mojave by close examination of the scales on the head. In the prairie rattler, the scales between the eyes on the top of the head are small and numerous, while on the Mojave, these scales are much larger and fewer. This is an admittedly difficult and usually unwise effort to undertake on a snake in the field! These snakes are often called "Mojave green rattlers" and indeed many specimens show an overall greenish cast. Others may be grayish, brownish, or yellowish. In my own experience those from the Big Bend region of west Texas are usually a greenish gray. One specimen I saw in Organ Pipe Cactus National Monument in southwestern Arizona was decidedly yellowish in color.

The food of the Mojave rattler as an adult consists mostly of small rodents that are plentiful in the desert. Young specimens also eat lizards that are another plentiful creature within this snake's habitat.

Though not as easily provoked as the western diamondback or even the prairie rattler, Mojaves are fairly high-strung snakes when encountered in the wild. After a short while in captivity, however, they become fairly docile. It should be stated that the keeping of venomous snakes in captivity by anyone other than a professional is usually unwise, and the potential for a tragic incident with a species like this cannot be overstated. All the reptile enthusiasts and curators that I know treat this snake with great respect. Among the victims of this snake's lethal bite was a professional involved in the study of snake venoms.

Recent efforts to produce a new, more effective antivenin for the treatment of pit viper bites has created a high demand for the venom of this rattlesnake. As a result, venom labs that provide the raw venom used in production of antivenin are working to obtain quantities of Mojave venom for sale to antivenin producers. One such venom lab operator, Jim Harrison of the Kentucky Reptile Zoo, has been collecting Mojaves for several years now and is poised to become a major contributor to this effort. Recently, while engaged in extracting venom from a number of these highly dangerous snakes, Jim experienced a near fatal bite from this species. Despite this incident and many other serious bites by other snakes over the years, he remains committed to his valuable work.

Black-Tailed Rattlesnake
(Crotalus molossus)
PHOTO #35 & 45 (right)

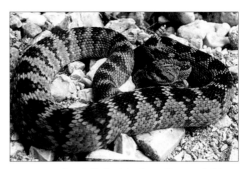

The black-tailed rattlesnake includes a total of three subspecies, only one of which, the northern black-tailed, is found in the United States. The other two subspecies, along with this one, range widely across northern Mexico. The range of our northern subspecies includes most of west Texas (including the Edwards Plateau and the Trans-Pecos region), extreme southern New Mexico, and much of Arizona (see range map).

As with most wide-ranging species, a fair amount of color variation occurs geographically, and there are two distinct color morphs of this snake in the United States. One, often referred to as the Texas phase (photo #35) is found in Texas, while the other, sometimes called Arizona phase (photo #45) ranges in New Mexico and Arizona. In some areas, solid black melanistic populations are known to exist. These melanistic individuals are found in the vicinity of ancient volcanoes where black lava (basalt) rocks are predominant. This tendency for coloration to match environmental conditions is a common phenomenon among many southwestern snake species. The advantage provided by blending in with the surroundings is obvious and is a good example of what biologists call "adaptive evolution."

Black-tailed rattlers are easily identified by the fact that they are the only rattlesnakes within their range with an all black tail and a black cap on the snout. They are medium size snakes that average about 3 feet in length as adults, but are capable of being larger — the record length being 4 feet 4 inches. Though not as dangerous as the larger eastern and western diamondbacks, timber/canebrakes, or the extremely venomous Mojave, the venom of the black-tailed does contain enzymes that, among other things, destroy the clotting ability of the blood, and a severe envenomation could prove fatal.

This snake is a habitat generalist, being found both on the desert flats and high into the mountains. On the desert floor they are a less common snake than

RANGE OF THE BLACK-TAILED RATTLESNAKE IN THE UNITED STATES

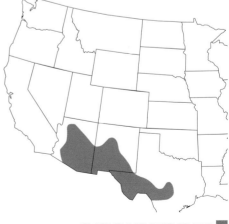

BLACK-TAILED RATTLESNAKE ■

many other rattlers within their range, but are more prevalent in mountains where they prefer canyons, rocky outcroppings and talus slopes. On one recent "herping" expedition, I found an individual prowling the desert floor at dusk in the Big Bend region of west Texas, and a few days later, located another coiled beneath a shelf of rock in Arizona's Chiricahua Mountains at an elevation of about 8,000 feet.

My own experience with this species confirms the general notion among herpetologists and reptile keepers that this is one of the more "laid back" rattlesnakes. I once collected one that, despite being pulled out from under a rock overhang with a snake hook and plunked unceremoniously into a bag, never rattled! On the other hand, I have seen them become thoroughly perturbed at such indignities and behave in a much more spirited fashion. Generally speaking, however, it is safe to say that these handsome snakes are less apt to strike in defense than most members of their clan. Interestingly, many snake hunters report seeing these snakes draped across the branches of shrubs and trees several feet off the ground. Their primary prey consists mostly of small mammals, with lizards also being eaten. Their occasional presence in arboreal situations suggests that baby birds may also be an important food item.

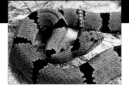

ROCK RATTLESNAKES
(Crotalus lepidus)

There are a total of four subspecies of this snake, but only two of which range northward into the United States from Mexico. In fact this is primarily a Mexican snake, and the two other subspecies are contained entirely in Mexico.

The name rock rattlesnake is very descriptive of these snakes as they are decidedly fond of rocks. They are most commonly found in rocky canyons and talus slopes, but may also be found in desert, arid grassland, and foothill slopes. They are usually associated with the arid land mountain ranges from west Texas through southern New Mexico to southeast Arizona, and southward into Mexico.

These are handsomely colored snakes that are highly variable in color. Their color and pattern varies to match the color of the rocks in the areas where they are found. They feed mostly on lizards, but also eat small rodents and amphibians. They are more diurnal than most rattlesnakes and are seemingly most active in the morning.

They are small snakes, averaging less than 2 feet in length. Their small size, tiny fangs, and small venom yields, make them less dangerous than many of the larger rattlesnakes; however, the venom of some specimens is quite potent and possesses a high percentage of neurotoxic components, probably an adaptation to their primarily cold-blooded diet of lizards and amphibians.

The reproduction rate for this species is low compared to most snakes, with only three to five young produced in an average litter. The babies resemble adults in color and pattern, but have the bright yellow tail tip seen in many other young pit vipers. A map depicting the approximate range of the two United States subspecies appears below, with accounts of the two races on the following page.

RANGE OF THE ROCK RATTLESNAKE IN THE UNITED STATES

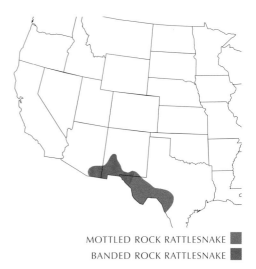

MOTTLED ROCK RATTLESNAKE ■
BANDED ROCK RATTLESNAKE ■

Mottled Rock Rattlesnake
(subspecies *lepidus*)
PHOTO #42

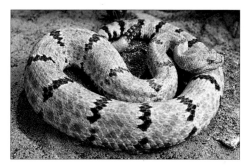

Like the related banded rattlesnake, the color of this snake mimics the color of the rocks in the area where they are found, and they are thus highly variable in color. Their overall color may be gray or bluish gray, often with a pink or purple hue. There are faint, dark bars that transverse the back and in the area between the bars there is a diffusion of dark pigments that produces a "mottled" effect.

This may be the only rattlesnake that has a non-venomous mimic in the form of the gray banded kingsnake (see photo #90). This harmless kingsnake shares its range with the mottled rock rattlesnake and mimics it closely enough to allow the assumption that it may obtain some benefit from the resemblance.

My experience with this snake in the wild is limited to a single encounter in the Big Bend National Park in Texas. While hiking in a picturesque canyon one morn-

ing in early August, I discovered an adult lying atop a large, flat-topped boulder about 6 feet above the ground. It was late morning and the temperature was already in the low 90s, but the boulder was still in the shade of the canyon wall. The snake perfectly matched the chalky gray of the boulder on which he was patiently waiting to ambush one of the many spiny lizards that were foraging throughout the canyon. They are mainly crepuscular and nocturnal in habits.

For additional reading on this subspecies see *Poisonous Snakes of Texas* and *A Field Guide to Texas Snakes* by Andrew Price or *Field Guide to the Snakes of Texas* by Alan Tennant.

Banded Rock Rattlesnake
(subspecies *klauberi*)
PHOTO #43 & 44 (right)

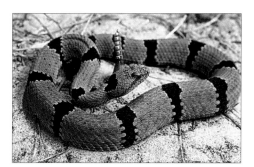

In this subspecies the dark transverse bars across the back are more pronounced than in the mottled rock, and there is little or no mottling between the bands. The result is a distinctly banded snake. The coloration on the body between the dark bands may be bluish-gray, bluish-green, purple or pink, making for an exceedingly beautifully colored little rattlesnake. As is the case with all rock rattlers, the color of this

race always matches the colors of the predominant rocks found in its habitat.

The range of the banded rock rattlesnake in the United States is contained mostly in Southern Arizona and southern

New Mexico, though they can also be found in the extreme western tip of Texas. Like many southwestern snakes, they are most active in early morning and late afternoon to early evening hours. Though essentially a montane snake, they are also found at lower elevations in the desert. I have hunted this attractive little rattler on a couple of occasions, but have not been fortunate enough to see one in the wild. Thus, all of the author's experiences with this snake have come from a few specimens kept in captivity.

The small size of these rattlesnakes equates to small venom glands and small amounts of venom. However, in some specimens the venom may be quite toxic. The Arizona Game & Fish publication, *The Venomous Reptiles of Arizona* by Lowe, Johnson, and Schwalbe, states that, "No humans have been killed, although occasionally bites have produced serious effects."

Twin-Spotted Rattlesnake
(Crotalus pricei)
PHOTO #41

This is one of a number of small montane rattlesnakes that inhabit isolated mountain ranges in the southwestern United States and Mexico. Among others are the rock rattlers and the ridge-nosed rattlers. Unlike the rock rattlers, which may sometimes be found at lower elevations, the twin-spotted is a snake of the higher peaks of desert mountains, trapped there eons ago when the climate changed and most of the area turned to desert, leaving them stranded on islands of mountaintops where the climate remained cool enough for these small rattlers.

Its color is a light gray with a paired row of dark spots down the back, a unique pattern among North American rattlesnakes. This little rattler is a true habitat specialist, existing only among the piles of talus that accumulate beneath high mountain peaks in the Chiricahua, Santa Rita, Huachuca, and Pinaleno Mountain ranges in Arizona. It may be found from 6,000 feet to beyond 10,000 feet in elevation. At these high altitudes,

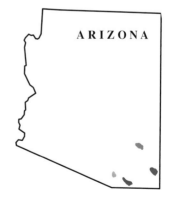

RANGE OF THE TWIN-SPOTTED RATTLESNAKE IN THE UNITED STATES

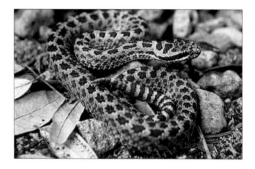

ARIZONA

PINALENO MOUNTAINS ■
CHIRICAHUA MOUNTAINS ■
HUACHUCA MOUNTAINS ■
SANTA CATALINA MOUNTAINS ■

the temperatures at which these cold-blooded reptiles are most comfortable occur during the day; thus this snake is basically a diurnal animal. Its primary prey is the mountain spiny lizard that shares its home among the rocks. It also eats mice, and captive specimens have persisted for years on mouse-only diets.

There are two subspecies of the twin-spotted rattlesnake, with the other subspecies limited to Mexico, which is the epicenter of distribution for this species. Its occurrence north of the Mexican border represents the northern limit of its range.

This is a dwarf rattlesnake, averaging less than 2 feet in length as an adult and reaching a maximum of 26 inches. They naturally have small fangs and their bite yields only small doses of venom, but the toxicity of their venom and the gravity of their bite to a human are unknown. Some very small rattlesnakes are known to possess a highly virulent venom (the midget faded for instance), and while it is doubtful that the twin-spotted is capable of inflicting a fatal bite, prudence dictates that such an event be treated with extreme caution. For most outdoorsmen, the risk of encountering this snake is so slight that any discussion of the danger of its bite is moot. They exist in so few places, and those places are so remote and out of the way that few people will ever venture into their realm.

I have visited the home of these little rattlers on the higher peaks of the Chiricahua Mountains, and while I did not see any, it was an interesting and insightful experience. To know that these rattlers can live in a place so alien to what most people regard as a good environment for snakes is a strong testimony to the adaptability and tenacity of the serpent, and a wonderful example of how these fascinating animals have evolved to occupy every available niche.

The author's only experience with this snake comes from a single captive specimen. In writing this account I have relied heavily on previously published material, especially the Arizona Game & Fish Publication *The Venomous Reptiles of Arizona*, by Lowe, Johnson, and Schwalbe. Due to their scarcity and limited range, these snakes are protected by the state of Arizona.

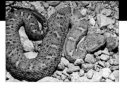

RIDGE-NOSED RATTLESNAKES
(Crotalus williardi)

The ridge-nosed rattlesnake has a total of five subspecies, only two of which range northward from Mexico into the United States. This species has much in common with the previously discussed rock rattlers and especially the twin-spotted rattler. First, it is primarily a Mexican species that ranges northward barely into the southwestern United States. Second, it is a rare, mountain snake found in isolated, remote mountain ranges surrounded by vast stretches of desert, which act as a barrier to its further distribution.

Very little is known of the natural history of this secretive species. They are known to feed on lizards, snakes, mice, and invertebrates including centipedes and scorpions. Babies are only about 7 inches long at birth and the litter size is small, averaging about four. Like many snakes found at higher elevations, they are thought to be strongly diurnal in habits. The name "ridge-nosed rattlesnake" comes from the pronounced ridge on the snout, and they are the only rattlesnakes to exhibit this characteristic. Though they are apparently not uncommon in suitable habitats, they are seemingly never abundant, and localities where they can be found are so few that they are protected by both state and federal wildlife agencies.

The toxicity of their venom is reputed to be low, and their small size (less than 2 feet) indicates that their bite is probably not deadly to humans. However, anyone bitten by this snake in its natural habitat would be many hours from medical care. Below is a map showing the range of the two subspecies native to the United States, and a brief account of each subspecies is on the following pages.

RANGE OF THE RIDGE-NOSED RATTLESNAKE IN THE UNITED STATES

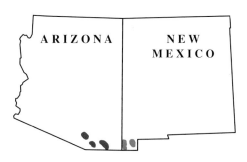

ARIZONA RIDGE-NOSED RATTLESNAKE ■
NEW MEXICO RIDGE-NOSED RATTLESNAKE ■

Arizona Ridge-Nosed Rattlesnake
(subspecies willardi)
PHOTO #47

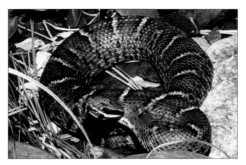

As its name implies, this race is found in Arizona. It may be found at elevations of 5,000 to 9,000 feet in the following desert mountain ranges near the Mexican border: the Huachuca, Santa Rita, and Patagonia Mountains. They reach a maximum length of 26.8 inches according to Carl Ernst in *Venomous Reptiles of North America.*

The Arizona ridge-nosed is told from the New Mexico ridge-nosed by the presence of pronounced white stripes on the side of the face and on the nose (see photo). This snake is a habitat specialist in the sense that it inhabits only desert mountains, but is a generalist in the sense that it occupies a number of microhabitats within its macrohabitat.

Concerns stemming from the potential for overcollecting of this subspecies by reptile enthusiasts has lead to their being protected by the state of Arizona.

At the time of this writing, the author has yet to encounter this snake in the wild, but a trip to its desert mountain home is a goal of every serious herpetologist, and a pilgrimage I hope to make soon. The specimen shown in photo #47 was photographed in captivity at the Birmingham Zoo.

New Mexico Ridge-Nosed Rattlesnake
(subspecies obscurus)
PHOTO #48

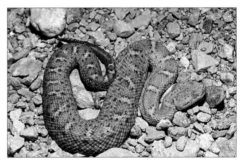

The Latin name *obscurus* refers to the coloration and pattern that on this subspecies are literally obscured. This is an almost uniformly gray or brownish snake with only a faint hint of a dorsal pattern. Additionally, the white stripes on the face that characterize all other races, including the Arizona ridge-nosed, are lacking. Its common name, New Mexico ridge-nosed, is also descriptive, as its range in the United States is restricted to two mountain ranges in extreme southwestern New Mexico. One of these mountain ranges, the Animas Mountains, is privately owned and access

to the area is restricted. The other desert mountain range where they are found, the southern Peloncillo Mountains, are federal lands but roads are few and access is difficult.

Because its restricted range in the United States makes it vulnerable to overcollecting by reptile enthusiasts, this subspecies of ridge-nosed rattler is regarded as a threatened species by the

U.S. Fish & Wildlife Service. The New Mexico Department of Game & Fish classifies it as endangered.

The author has visited the haunts of this snake in the Peloncillo Mountains, and though the area is remote and difficult to access, serious snake collectors are undaunted by such challenges and it is probably for the best that the snake is protected. Like many naturalists, the author revels in trekking to such rarely visited places to observe a fauna seen in its natural habitat by so few.

These small, secretive mountain rattlers reach a maximum length of 25 inches. For more details on their natural history see the species account. For additional reading on this snake, refer to *Amphibians and Reptiles of New Mexico* by Degenhardt, Painter, and Price.

Tiger Rattlesnake
(Crotalus tigris)
PHOTO #46

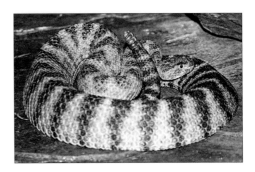

The range of the tiger rattlesnake in the United States is contained within the Sonoran Desert region of south-central Arizona, where it associates with rocky situations among desert foothills. Its range extends southward from Arizona for some distance into Mexico.

Both the common and scientific names derive from the distinctly banded pattern of "tiger stripes" that are apparent down the entire length of the body. The color of this snake is highly variable, ranging from pinkish or reddish to bluish gray or yellowish brown. As with many other desert rattlesnakes, the color tends to match the colors of the rocks present in the snake's environment.

The tiger rattlesnake is sometimes confused with the speckled rattlesnake, as both exhibit a dorsal pattern of bands rather than blotches. The tiger rattler may be readily distinguished from the speckled rattlesnake (which has three subspecies) by its exceptionally small head. In proportion to body size, the tiger rattlesnake has the smallest head of any rat-

**RANGE OF THE
TIGER RATTLESNAKE
IN THE UNITED STATES**

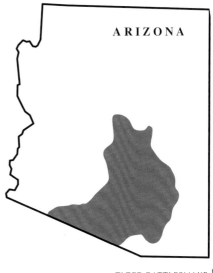

ARIZONA

TIGER RATTLESNAKE ▪

tlesnake species. The small head is thought to be an adaptation for feeding on lizards, which overnight in the many rock crevices that abound in the tiger rattler's habitat of rocky canyons, outcrops, and talus. Hunting after dark when the diurnal lizards have taken refuge within the rock crevices, the tiger rattler's small head allows it to search for its prey deep within narrow cracks where larger predators are unable to reach. Though lizards are probably a staple food source, they are also known to eat mice, and on rare occasions they have been observed climbing into low bushes that may indicate predation of bird's nests.

These are smallish rattlesnakes, averaging about 2 to 2½ feet in length with a maximum length of about 3 feet. Due to their exceptionally small head, tiger rattlesnakes have smaller venom glands and are capable of injecting only small amounts of venom. However, the venom is quite toxic, containing a high amount of neurotoxins and on a drop-for-drop basis, it may be one of the most toxic of the rattlesnakes. Thus, it would appear that despite its low venom yield, there is a potential for this snake to be deadly to humans, and most experts express extreme caution in dealing with this snake. In contrast, Carl Ernst in his book *Venomous Reptiles of North America* concludes (after citing a number of venom studies), "Tiger Rattlesnake envenomation of humans produces little local reaction and no significant systemic symptoms."

Baby tigers, which are miniature replicas of the adults, have such tiny heads that the only vertebrate prey available would seem to be young lizards. These snakes have a peak activity period that coincides with the seasonal rains, or monsoons, that occur in the desert in late summer. It is during this time that most tiger rattlesnakes are observed and/or collected by herpetologists.

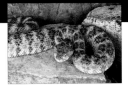

SPECKLED RATTLESNAKES
(Crotalus mitchelli)

This rattlesnake is represented by a total of five subspecies, two of which are found in the southwestern United States, a third in Baja, Mexico, and two others that are restricted to off-shore islands in the Sea of Cortéz. In appearance it is somewhat similar to the tiger rattlesnake, in that it exhibits a banded pattern that is uncommon on rattlesnakes in the southwestern United States. The coloration of this species is extremely variable, depending on the color of the rocks and gravel where the individual snake lives. A diffusion of small speckles gives a "salt and pepper" effect to its overall appearance, and on most specimens a distinct banding occurs on the distal portion of the body.

These are decidedly desert snakes, being found in both the Mojave and Sonoran Deserts. They may range from the desert floor up into the foothills of desert mountain ranges. They feed mostly on warm-blooded prey like the kangaroo rat, which is exceedingly common throughout their range. Other small mammals are also eaten along with lizards that are probably the primary food for the young. Like all pit vipers, the young are born alive. Litters may number from two or three for young females to 10 or 11 in large females in their prime.

This is a medium large species that can exceed 4 feet in length and its venom is reported to be quite toxic, leading to the conclusion that it is capable of inflicting a fatal bite. The range for the two United States subspecies is shown on the map below with accounts of the two subspecies on the following pages.

RANGE OF THE SPECKLED RATTLESNAKE IN THE UNITED STATES

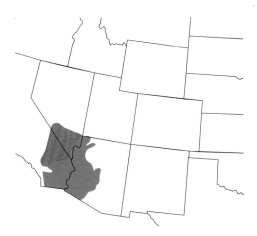

PANAMINT RATTLESNAKE ■
SOUTHWESTERN SPECKLED RATTLESNAKE ■

Panamint Rattlesnake

(subspecies *stephensi*)

PHOTO #54

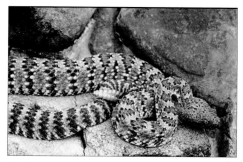

This race of speckled rattlesnake gets its name from the Panamint Mountains of Death Valley, California. Its range also includes the entire Mojave Desert region of southernmost Nevada and southwestern California, being replaced by its cousin the southwestern speckled rattler in the Sonoran Desert region (see range map). Distinguishing between the races of *Crotalus mitchelli* is difficult, since both are extremely variable in color. Herpetologists rely on a close examination of certain scales on the snout and above the eye to make certain identification, but the easiest (and safest) way to determine which subspecies you are dealing with is to know the location where the specimen was found.

These are extremely variable snakes in color, with the color matching the substrate of the snake's environment almost precisely. Most specimens of the Panamint rattler I have seen resemble the specimen pictured in photo #54, which I photographed in the Panamint Mountains of Death Valley, one of the hottest and driest places on earth and an exceptionally harsh environment to which these snakes seem quite well suited.

This race is somewhat smaller than others of its species, and rarely exceeds 3 feet. This subspecies is fairly docile in nature, and usually not too quick to defend, a somewhat puzzling behavior since its larger cousin the southwestern speckled rattler is known for its irritability. The bite of this snake, however, is a serious affair as their venom may be quite toxic and they are presumably capable of killing. For additional information on the biology of this snake, see the species account for *crotalus mitchelli*.

Southwestern Speckled Rattlesnake

(subspecies *pyrrhus*)

PHOTO #53

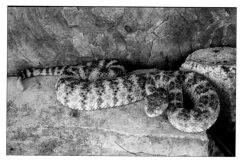

If anything, this race of the speckled rattler is even more variable in color than the preceding form (Panamint). In fact, it is generally regarded as being the most inconsistently colored of any rattlesnake, and as with its cousin the Panamint, the colors always match exactly the colors of the rocks, gravel, or sand where the snake is found. The basic pattern of heavily diffused speckling is always present, and even wildly different color morphs are recognizable as being *c. mitchelli* by experienced herpetologists.

These snakes will match their surroundings so well that their camouflaging effect makes them almost impossible to see when not moving. This fact can lead to an unfortunate encounter for the outdoorsman, as they are easily provoked and fairly quick to strike when threatened. The venom of this snake may vary from one geographic area to another, with some specimens being quite potent, and they are capable of injecting a fairly large amount in their strike; thus, they should be considered quite capable of killing.

This subspecies of speckled rattler is a snake of the Sonoran Desert region of southwestern Arizona and southeastern California. It also ranges southward well down into Mexico's Baja peninsula. Throughout its range, its favorite haunts are rocky areas that afford it easy access to cover. When fully grown, the southwestern speckled rattlesnake may slightly exceed 4 feet in length, with an absolute maximum of 4 feet 5 inches being recorded. Additional information on the natural history of this subspecies is contained in the species account.

Red Diamond Rattlesnake

(Crotalus ruberi)

PHOTO #64

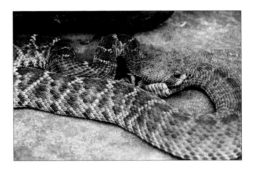

This is another one of the "big three" diamondback rattlers found in the United States; the other two being the eastern diamondback and the western diamondback. This snake exhibits the classic diamond-shaped blotches that characterize the diamondbacks, but its overall color is decidedly reddish, hence its name. In size, it is one of our largest rattlesnake species, with most adults reaching a length of 4 to 5 feet. The record length of 5 feet 5 inches puts it in fourth place among North American rattlesnakes. It is also a rather stout, heavy-bodied snake.

These snakes have a limited range in the United States, being found only in southernmost California where they are still fairly common in some areas. Here, they are found mostly within the natural region known as the "peninsular ranges," which are mountain ranges that extend

**RANGE OF THE
RED DIAMOND RATTLESNAKE
IN THE UNITED STATES**

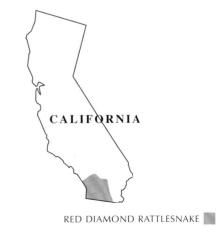

CALIFORNIA

RED DIAMOND RATTLESNAKE ▪

northward from the Baja peninsula of Mexico. They may be found in suitable habitats from sea level to near 5,000 feet in elevation. They range southward well into Baja, where at least two other sub-species can be found, one in the southern tip of the peninsula and one on a Pacific island off the coast. Robert Stebbins in his classic *Peterson Field Guide to Western Reptiles and Amphibians* writes of this snake's habitat, "Frequents desert scrub, thorn scrub, open chaparral, and woodland; occasionally also found in grassland and cultivated areas." While Carl Ernst in *Venomous Reptiles of North America* writes that it "is most common in the western foothills of the coastal ranges, but also lives in dry, rocky, inland valleys."

Like many larger snake species, red diamond rattlers are capable of producing large litters numbering up to 20, with about half that number being the average litter size. Youngsters resemble the adults, but are less reddish and tend to be grayish in color at first, gradually becoming redder with age. The babies are quite large, averaging just over a foot in length at birth.

These rattlesnakes as adults feed mostly on mammals, including such animals as kangaroo and wood rats and ground squirrels. The larger adults are quite capable of swallowing a full-grown cottontail rabbit. They are also known to eat birds occasionally, and lizards are apparently an important food source for the young. Hybridization with the Southern Pacific rattlesnake has been known to occur in the wild.

The large size and subsequently large venom glands make this snake a potentially deadly animal to man. However, its venom drop for drop is not nearly as toxic as with many other rattlesnakes, and its temperament is mild, making it considerably less dangerous than America's other two diamondbacks. The author's only experience with this species has come from captive specimens, which I found to be exceedingly mild mannered.

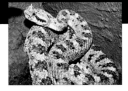

SIDEWINDER RATTLESNAKES
(Crotalus cerastes)

There are three very similar sub-species of sidewinder rattlesnakes found in the United States. They are so much alike that positive identification down to the subspecies level is difficult even for experts. For most people, the only way to be absolutely sure to which subspecies a specimen belongs is to know the locality where it was found.

Their name comes from their peculiar "side-winding" form of locomotion, which entails moving by elevating a loop of the body and advancing it forward, pressing the loop down and using it as an anchor while elevating and advancing forward another portion of the body. This method is particularly well suited to moving across loose sand, which is common in much of their habitat, and they are capable of surprising speed when using this method. Another advantage gained by using this method is that it keeps most of the snake's body off the hot desert floor, an important consideration for an ectothermic creature that can quickly succumb to overheating.

Sidewinders are desert specialists, being found only in the Sonoran and Mojave Desert regions. They are most common where the substrate is sandy and vegetation is sparse. As with most desert dwellers, they are primarily nocturnal in habits and escape the heat of the day by entering rodent burrows or by burying themselves in the sand. Above each eye is a raised scale that apparently is an adaptation that somehow protects and/or shades the eye. Another possible function is to help trap and hold sand on the top of the head so a buried snake can hold the head nearer the surface to maintain vision with eyes just above sand. The trapped sand on the top of the head not only hides the snake, but shields it from the blazing sun as well.

Other desert-dwelling snakes in other parts of the world, like the desert horned viper of North Africa and the Arabian

RANGE OF THE SIDEWINDER RATTLESNAKE IN THE UNITED STATES

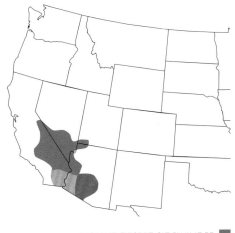

MOJAVE DESERT SIDEWINDER ■
SONORAN DESERT SIDEWINDER ■
COLORADO DESERT SIDEWINDER ■

Peninsula, also show the same special adaptations for existing in hot, sandy environments. The horned viper uses the sidewinding locomotion and also possesses specialized raised scales above the eye. The two snakes are completely unrelated and live on opposite sides of the globe but are morphologically and behaviorally very similar. This is a classic example of what biologists term "convergent evolution."

In color the sidewinders are always some shade of pale brown or tan, often with a yellowish, reddish, or grayish hue, but blending well with the color of the sand in their habitat. There is a series of slightly darker dorsal blotches that create a cryptic "pebbled" effect.

These are small snakes, averaging about 18 to 20 inches in length as adults, and reaching a maximum of 33 inches. Their venom is fairly toxic but they are capable of injecting only a small dose, and they are generally not considered as dangerous to man as many other rattlesnakes. Still, there is the potential for a fatal bite. The prey of these small rattlers consists of rodents, lizards, and birds.

The following accounts of the three subspecies are limited to identification only, as the natural history of these snakes is essentially the same. Identification methods involve counting the number of scale rows present at mid-body (not an option for most casual observers) and noting the color of the basal (first) segment of the rattle. While the author is usually inclined to support the concept of subspecies (see comments on timber/canebrake rattlers), in this case the argument for subspecific status seems weak. As stated in the opening paragraph, the surest way to determine the subspecies of this snake is to know the locality where it was found (see range map on the previous page).

Mojave Desert Sidewinder

(subspecies *cerastes*)

PHOTO #50

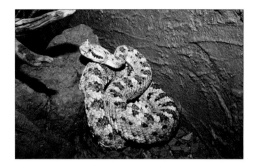

As its name implies, this subspecies inhabits the Mojave Desert. It is the most northerly of the three subspecies and ranges all the way up into east-central California, southern Nevada, and a small portion of southwestern Utah. This race is identified by the brown color of the basal segment of the rattle, and the 21 rows of scales at mid-body.

Sonoran Desert Sidewinder

(subspecies *cercobombus*)

PHOTO #51

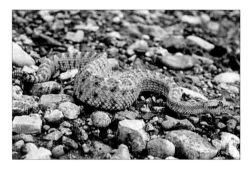

Found in the Sonoran Desert region of central Arizona, southward into Sonora, Mexico, this subspecies is identified by the black basal rattle segment and 21 rows of scales at mid-body.

Colorado Desert Sidewinder

(subspecies *laterorepens*)

PHOTO #52

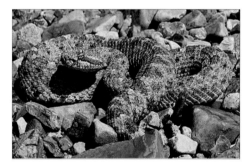

The range of this subspecies includes extreme southeastern California and southwestern Arizona, then southward into northern Baja, Mexico. This region is known as the Colorado Desert area, which is a sub-division of the larger Sonoran Desert region. This subspecies is distinguished from the other two races by its black basal rattle segment and 23 scale rows at mid-body.

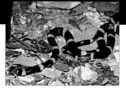

EASTERN CORAL SNAKES
(Micrurus fulvius)

Coral snakes are one of the most easily recognized of snakes, being brightly colored with alternate rings of red, yellow, and black. This color pattern has been mimicked by a number of other snakes, especially the Florida Scarlet Snake and the Scarlet Kingsnake (see photos #79 and #80). See also the drawings on page 17.

According to outdoor folklore, all coral snakes are tiny snakes with jaws so small that they can bite a human only on the webbing between the fingers or on the ear lobes. Not so! Though coral snakes are much smaller than most pit vipers, possessing less well-developed venom delivery systems, and are docile and shy, an enraged adult coral snake can give a good account of itself in its ability to bite a human. They are, however, normally reluctant to bite, and the late Ross Allen related to the author an instance where he encountered a small child walking down the street in Ocala, Florida, with an Eastern Coral Snake in his hand. Ross relieved the youth of his dangerous pet without either of them being bitten. In contrast, I have seen agitated coral snakes bite and chew deliberately on their water bowl or the floor of their cage after being subjected to the indignities of being handled by their keepers for a venom extraction.

Drop for drop, the venom of the coral snakes is among the most toxic animal venoms known, and in the very few cases where substantial envenomation occurs; specific coral snake antivenin is the only effective treatment. Unlike the bites of pit vipers, coral snake envenomations may not show pronounced symptoms for several hours after the bite. Once symptoms begin to appear, however, they can be difficult to reverse. For this reason, any bite by a coral snake should be treated aggressively, and the administration of antivenin should be considered, even if obvious symptoms are lacking.

Coral snakes are members of the family Elapidae, or cobra family, and their venom is entirely neurotoxic,

RANGE OF THE EASTERN CORAL SNAKES IN THE UNITED STATES

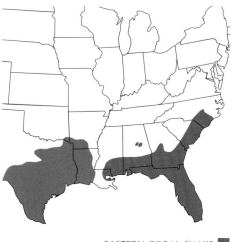

EASTERN CORAL SNAKE ■
TEXAS CORAL SNAKE ■

attacking nerve endings and killing by blocking nerve impulses, resulting in paralysis of the diaphragm. A third member of the Elapidae family, the Arizona Coral Snake, genus *Micruroides* is also found in the United States.

These are small-headed, slim-bodied snakes that average about 2½ to 3 feet in length. The recognized record length for this snake is given as 47¾ inches in *Peterson Field Guide to Reptiles and Amphibians of Eastern/Central North America* by Conant and Collins. Other experts (Tennant and Bartlett in *Snakes of North America:Eastern and Central Regions*) give the record length as 51 inches. I was fortunate enough to spend a number of years in the heart of Eastern coral snake country in Marion County, Florida, in the early 1970s and saw a number of specimens over 40 inches in length. During this same time period, I helped measure a 49-inch specimen that was brought to the venom lab at the Ross Allen Reptile Institute.

Unlike the pit vipers that give birth to fully formed young, coral snakes are egg layers. A typical clutch may include six to eight eggs, with the maximum being about a dozen. The hatchlings are miniature replicas of the adults but quite tiny, being only 6 inches in length and no bigger around than an earthworm.

Much has been written over the years regarding the bright colors of dangerous animals like the Coral Snakes and the species that mimic them. The widely held belief is that the bright colors act as a warning to potential predators, and that species that mimic this warning gain a degree of protection. Since most potential mammalian predators of this snake are color blind, and are mostly nocturnally active, some scientists have suggested that the coral snake's colors are meant to protect them against the diurnal birds of prey which have good color vision. The disruptive nature of the alternate brightly colored rings has also been cited as having a cryptic effect by breaking up the snake's outline. Less well known is what I call the "confusion factor" created when the snake is crawling. I experienced this phenomenon myself on one occasion in the Ocala National Forest. While I was hiking on a trail through a palmetto thicket, a coral snake suddenly crawled across my trail. The first sensation I had was one of a stationary object flashing bright red and yellow in the path. By the time I was able to bring the snake into focus, its tail was disappearing into the palmetto.

Adult coral snakes feed on lizards and other snakes. Young snakes probably feed mostly on invertebrates. Coral snakes are known to curl and raise the end to their tail when threatened. This interesting behavior parallels the rattle of rattlesnakes and the tail shaking of many other snake species as a method of detracting attention from the vulnerable anterior of a snake to the least vulnerable tail.

There are two subspecies of *Micrurus fulvius* in the United States; both are alike in habits and habitat, and their physical differences are so slight that this author questions the validity of subspecific status for this snake.* The range map on the opposite page shows the approximate range of the two subspecies, and a brief description of both is on the following page.

* Recent studies conducted since the original publication of this volume have resulted in herpetologists regarding the two as distinct species.

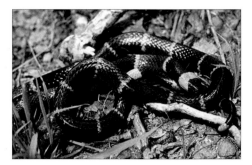

Eastern Coral Snake
(subspecies *fulvius*)
PHOTO #17

The Eastern Coral Snake may be differentiated from the Texas Coral Snake by the fact that there is much less black spotting diffused within the red bands. On some specimens in the southern Florida peninsula, the red bands are entirely lacking of black pigment and are much broader in width. For more data on this snake, read "Eastern Coral Snakes" on the preceding pages.

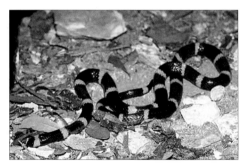

Texas Coral Snake
(subspecies *tenere*)
PHOTO #18

The Texas Coral Snake differs from the eastern subspecies in that there is a large amount of black spotting present within the red bands, with a resultant much darker appearance of the snake. Despite the name Texas Coral Snake, this race is also found in much of Louisiana and a small area of southern Arkansas. See the range map and the account for the Eastern Coral Snakes on the preceding pages for additional information.

Western Coral Snake
(Micruroides euryxanthus)
PHOTO #37

This is primarily a Mexican species which has a total of three subspecies, one of which *(euryxanthus)* ranges into the southwestern United States in southern Arizona and southwestern New Mexico. In color and pattern, they are very much like the Eastern Corals, exhibiting the classic red, black, and yellow rings around the body. In this species, however, the yellow rings may be cream or nearly white. They are smaller than their eastern counterparts, averaging only about 14 inches in length. The record length is 24^1/$_2$ inches. In girth, the largest individuals may reach the diameter of a pencil.

These diminutive members of the cobra family feed mostly on small lizards and snakes, especially the fossorial (burrowing) blind snakes (genus *Leptotyphlops*) that are the tiniest snakes in America, being no larger than an average size earthworm. Western Corals are confirmed burrowers and spend much of their time underground. They are thus only rarely encountered by humans.

Though their venom is quite potent, they are generally not inclined to bite and are capable of injecting only small amounts of venom. There have been no deaths recorded from their bite. Though they may be capable of killing, the threat these snakes pose to the average outdoorsman is negligible.

Like the Eastern Coral Snakes,

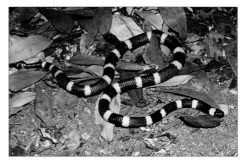

Western Corals have some well-known mimics among harmless snake species, most notably the Sonoran Shovel Nosed Snake (photo #96) and the Arizona Mountain Kingsnake (photo #89).

The approximate range for this species in the United States is shown on map below.

RANGE OF THE WESTERN CORAL SNAKE IN THE UNITED STATES

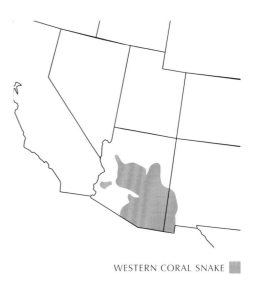

WESTERN CORAL SNAKE

GLOSSARY

Acclimate — to adjust or become tolerant of a new or different climate.

Adaptation — change that takes place in structure, function, or behavior in adjusting to a new condition or environment.

Adaptive evolution — evolving to adapt to a particular environment.

Amphibian — a class of vertebrate animals that includes frogs, toads, salamanders, and the little known caecilians.

Anteriorly — toward the head.

Antivenin — antibody or antitoxin administered to snakebite victims to neutralize the effects of envenomation. Most antivenin produced today is made from the blood of horses that have been repeatedly injected with gradually increasing doses of a mixture of snake venoms. The blood contains molecules known as antibodies, which when injected into a snakebite victim bind with molecules of venom and render it harmless. Also called antivenom.

Appalachian Mountains — a more or less continuous chain of mountain ranges in the eastern United States, which runs from Maine to northern Georgia and extreme northeastern Alabama, and including several smaller mountain ranges, the best known of which are the Smoky Mountains, the Adirondack Mountains, the Blue Ridge Mountains, the Catskill Mountains, and the White Mountains.

Arboreal — pertaining to trees..

Arid — dry

Atypical — not typical, unusual.

Basal — at the beginning or base.

Biology — all the traits, behaviors, and physical characteristics associated with a living organism. Also the science of the study of life.

Biome — a community of plants and animals that characterize a particular type of habitat, such as desert, tundra, woodland, etc.

Buteo — a genus of hawks characterized by their broad wings and soaring habits.

Carnivore — a flesh eater.

Carrion — a dead animal.

Caudal — pertaining to the tail.

Chaparral — vegetation consisting of thickets of dwarfed, drought-tolerant shrubs and bushes.

Chihuahuan Desert — North America's largest desert region, contained mostly in Mexico but including west Texas, much of southern New Mexico, and a tiny area of southeast Arizona.

Cline (or clinal) — A gradual change in physical characteristics (such as color) in a population of animals over a wide geographical area in which individuals from the two extremes are markedly different.

Coastal Plain — a geophysical province of the southeastern United States that begins at the seashore and extends inland to upland areas. Generally flat with only small amounts of relief in the form of erosion of low hills or ridges.

Colorado Desert — a subdivision of the Sonoran Desert contained in southwestern Arizona and southeastern California.

Communal — living together.

Contiguous — adjoining, adjacent to, in contact with.

Convergent evolution — the tendency of unrelated animals in a particular habitat to acquire similar adaptive structures.

Crepuscular — pertaining to twilight, active at dawn or dusk.

Crotalid — a pit viper (rattlesnake, copperhead, cottonmouth).

Cryptic — hidden or concealed. Adapted for concealment.

Cumberland Plateau — an area of upland drained by the Cumberland and Kentucky Rivers, including parts of the southern Appalachian Mountains. Includes much of eastern Kentucky, eastern Tennessee, western Virginia, and northern Alabama.

Deciduous — trees and plants which shed their leaves each winter.

Disjunct — not connected to others, separated from.

Distal — away from; in animals usually means from the head, toward the tail.

Diurnal — pertaining to daytime, active during the day.

Docile — tame.

Ectothermic — cold blooded, refers to animals which are unable to regulate body temperature internally, i.e., reptiles, amphibians, fishes, etc.

Elapidae — family of snakes characterized by short, immovable fangs and a primarily neurotoxic venom, often called the cobra family.

Elapid — a member of the snake family Elapidae.

Elliptical — shaped like and ellipse, oval shaped.

Envenomation — to inject venom or have venom injected.

Flint Hills — a geophysical province in east-central Kansas characterized by mostly treeless tall grass prairie with numerous rocky outcroppings of limestone and flint.

Fossorial — burrowing.

Genera — plural of genus.

Genus — a subdivision of a family of animals consisting of one or more related species.

Habitat — the natural home of an organism.

Hemorrhagic — to cause bleeding, often internally.

Herpetologist — one who studies the science of herpetology.

Herpetology — the science of the study of reptiles and amphibians.

Herping — a slang word for the act of hunting reptiles and amphibians.

Hibernacula — a site for hibernation, usually underground.

Hibernate or hibernation — to pass the winter in a dormant or lethargic state.

Hybrid — an offspring resulting from the crossbreeding of two different species.

Hybridize — to produce a hybrid.

Immune; immunity — not susceptible to.

Intergradation — the melding of characters of two or more subspecies within a population of animals.

Intergrade — an offspring resulting from the crossbreeding of two different subspecies, or a population of animals that exhibits characters intermediate between two or more subspecies.

Invertebrate — an animal which lacks a backbone, as in crustaceans, insects, arachnids, etc.

Macrohabitat — a large area of habitat such as "pine forest" or "desert flats".

Microhabitat — a small area of habitat contained within the larger macrohabitat; examples would be "talus slope"(micro) in "desert mountain ranges"(macro).

Mimic — to appear like, to imitate.

Mississippi Delta — a region of lands on each side of the lower Mississippi River that are subject to or have been subject to flooding of the Mississippi River.

Mixed grass prairie — a transitional zone between the short grass prairies of the western great plains and the tall grass prairies of the East, containing both short and tall grass plant species.

Mogollon Rim — an area of mountainous highlands consisting mostly of coniferous forests that run diagonally across Arizona from northwest to southeast, extending into west-central New Mexico.

Mojave Desert — a desert region that covers southern Nevada and much of southwest and south-central California.

Montane — pertaining to plants and animals of the mountains.

Morphologically — pertaining to morphology, i.e., the physical form, color, etc. ,of an organism.

Natural history — the entire nature of an organism, i.e., its habitat, adaptations, behaviors, reproduction, etc. Also the study of nature.

Necrosis — the death of living tissue.

Neurotoxic and neurotoxins — toxic or poisonous to nerve cells and tissues; disruptive to the function and physiology of nerve cells or tissues.

Niche — the place or position occupied by an organism in the overall ecology.

Nocturnal — pertaining to night; active at night.

Olfactory — pertaining to the sense of smell.

Ozark Plateau and Ozarks — the mountainous areas and surrounding highlands of Missouri and northern Arkansas, characterized by a predominance of oak/hickory forests and cedar glades.

Phylogeny (phylogenetic) — pertaining to ancestral development.

Physiological (physiologically) — pertaining to the various processes, activities, and functions of living tissue.

Pit viper — any venomous snake of the family Crotalidae, characterized by movable, erectable fangs and the presence of a pit on the side of the face containing a heat-sensory organ.

Race — see subspecies.

Raptor — a bird of prey (hawk, owl, eagle, falcon).

Raptorial — pertaining to a raptor or bird of prey.

Relict — a survivor or remnant of a once flourishing group.

Rhomboid — a shape consisting of four sides, more or less an irregular square.

Short grass prairie — grasslands characterized by grasses less than 2 feet in height and occurring along the eastern slope of the Rocky Mountains where the "rain shadow" effect of the mountains creates an area of limited rainfall.

Sonoran Desert — a large desert region that covers much of northwestern Mexico (including the Baja peninsula), southern Arizona, and extreme southeastern California.

Species — a subdivision of a genus consisting of a group of individuals with a common ancestry, that closely resemble each other and in nature interbreed and produce fertile offspring.

Subspecies — a subdivision of a species consisting of a group of individuals, usually a geographic race, that differs slightly from other groups (subspecies) of the same species but between which interbreeding is possible. In this book; the terms subspecies and race are used interchangeably.

Substrate — the soil, rock, sand, etc., upon which an organism lives.

Sympatrically — occurring in the same or overlapping areas.

Systemic — pertaining to or affecting organ systems.

Tall grass prairie — the generally flat geographic region once dominated by tall grasses (i.e. big bluestem, Indian grass, Switch Grass, etc.), includes all of the Corn Belt and much of the Midwest.

Talus — an accumulation of rocks or boulders constituting fragments of a mountain, which accumulate beneath cliffs and peaks.

Terrestrial — pertaining to the earth, a ground-dwelling organism.

Trans Pecos — a region of west Texas, west and south of the Pecos River.

Tympanic membrane — the eardrum.

Venom — a toxic substance produced by animals.

Xeric — pertaining to arid or dry conditions.

REFERENCES
Books

Ashton, R.E. and P.S. Ashton. *Handbook of Reptiles and Amphibians of Florida, Part 1, The Snakes.* Miami: Windward Publishing, 1981.

Bartlett, R.D. and Alan Tennant. *Snakes of North America Western Region.* Houston, Texas: Gulf Publishing Co., 2000.

Baxter, G.T. and M.D. Stone. *Amphibians and Reptiles of Wyoming.* Cheyenne: Wyoming Game and Fish Department, 1985.

Brown, H.A., R.B. Bruce, D.M. Darda, L.V. Diller, C.R. Peterson, and R.M. Storm. *Reptiles of Washington and Oregon.* Seattle, Washington: Seattle Audubon Society, 1995.

Brown, Phillip R. *A Field Guide to the Snakes of California.* Houston, Texas: Gulf Publishing Co., 1997.

Collins, Joseph T. *Amphibians and Reptiles in Kansas.*Lawrence, Kansas: University Press of Kansas, 1993.

Conant, R. and J.T. Collins. *Peterson Field Guide to Reptiles and Amphibians of Eastern/Central North America.* New York: Houghton Mifflin Co., 1998.

Christiansen, J.L. and Reeve M. Bailey. *The Snakes of Iowa.* Des Moines, Iowa: Iowa Conservation Commission, 1992.

Degenhardt, W.G., C.W. Painter, and A.H. Price. *Amphibeans and Reptiles of New Mexico.* Albuquerque, New Mexico: University of New Mexico Press, 1996.

Ditmars, Raymond L. *The Reptiles of North America.* Garden City, New York: Doubleday & Co. Inc., 1936.

Ernst, Carl H. *Venomous Reptiles of North America.* Washington, DC: Smithsonian Institution Press, 1992.

Hammerson, Geoffrey A. *Amphibians and Reptiles in Colorado.* Denver: Colorado Division of Wildlife, 1986.

Johnson, Tom R. *The Amphibians and Reptiles of Missouri.* Jefferson City, Missouri: Missouri Department of Conservation, 1987.

Klauber, Lawrence M. *Rattlesnakes: Their Habits, Life Histories, and Influence on Mankind.* Berkely: University of California Press, 1982.

Levell, John P. *A Field Guide to Reptiles and Amphibians and the Law.* Excelsior, Minnesota: Serpents Tale, 1995.

Lowe, C.H. T.B. Johnson, and C.R Schwalbe. *The Venomous Reptiles of Arizona.* Pheonix: Arizona Game and Fish Department, 1986.

Minton, S.A. and M.R. Minton. *Venomous Reptiles. New York:*Charles Scribner & Sons, 1969.

Mitchell, J. C. *The Reptiles of Virginia.*Washington, D.C.:Smithsonian Institution Press, 1994.

Mount, Robert H. *The Reptiles and Amphibians of Alabama.*Auburn, Alabama: Alabama University, Press, 1975.

Palmer, W.M. and A. L. Braswell. *Reptiles of North Carolina.* Chapel Hill: University of North Carolina Press, 1995.

Phillips, C.A., R..A. Brandon, and E.O. Moll. *Field Guide to Amphibians and Reptiles in Illinois.* Champaign: Illinois Natural History Survey, 1999.

Price, Andrew H. *Poisonous Snakes of Texas.* Austin: Texas Parks and Wildlife, 1998.

Oldfield, B. and J.J. Moriaty. *Amphibians and Reptiles Native to Minnesota.* Minneapolis: University of Minnesota Press, 1994.

Stebbins, Robert C. *Peterson Field Guide to Western Reptiles and Amphibians. New York:* Houghton Mifflin Co., 1985.

Tennant, Alan. *A Field Guide to the Snakes of Florida.* Houston: Gulf Publishing Co., 1997.

Tennant, Alan, and R.D. Bartlett. *Snakes of North America: Eastern and Central Regions.* Houston: Gulf Publishing Co., 2000.

Tennant, Alan, J.E. Werhler., and B. Marvell. *A Field Guide to Texas Snakes.* Houston: Gulf Publishing Co., 1985.

Williamson, M. A., P.W. Hyder, and J.S. Applegart. *Snakes, Lizards, Turtles, Frogs, Toads, and Salamanders of New Mexico.* Sante Fe, New Mexico: Sunstone Press, 1994.

Wright, A.H. and Anna Allen Wright. *Handbook of Snakes of the United States and Canada .*Ithaca, New York: Comstock Publishing Associates, 1957.

INDEX